Mindfulness-Related Treatments and Addiction Recovery

While mindfulness meditation has been used in clinical settings as an adjunctive treatment for substance use disorders for some time, there has been limited empirical evidence to support this practice. *Mindfulness-Related Treatments and Addiction Recovery* bridges this gap by reporting the findings of studies in which mindfulness practice has been combined with other behavioural treatments and/or adapted to meet the needs of a variety of client populations in recovery. Therapies used as interventions in the described studies include Mindfulness-Based Stress Reduction (MBSR), Mindfulness-Based Cognitive Therapy (MBCT), Dialectical Behavior Therapy (DBT), Acceptance and Commitment Therapy (ACT), Mindfulness-Based Relapse Prevention (MBRP), and Mindfulness-Based Therapeutic Community (MBTC) treatment. This book offers a glimpse into the many ways in which mindfulness strategies have been applied to various facets of the recovery process including stress, craving, anxiety, and other relapse related factors. Preliminary evidence, while not conclusive, suggests that mindfulness-based therapies are effective, safe, satisfying to clients, and that an individual, at-home mindfulness practice can be potentially sustained over time, beyond the intervention duration.

This book was originally published as two volumes of the journal *Substance Abuse*.

Marianne T. Marcus, EdD, RN, FAAN is the John P. McGovern Distinguished Professor of Addiction Nursing and Director of the Center of Substance Abuse Education, Prevention and Research at the University of Texas Health Science Center at Houston School of Nursing. Her research area is mindfulness in therapeutic community settings.

Aleksandra Zgierska, MD, PhD is an Assistant Professor at the Department of Family Medicine, School of Medicine and Public Health, University of Wisconsin-Madison. Stemming from her active clinical practice in family medicine and addiction medicine, her research focuses on innovative therapies, especially mindfulness-based interventions, for addictive disorders.

This book is dedicated to G. Alan Marlatt, PhD (November 26, 1941–March 14, 2011) – a wonderful friend, colleague, caring clinician, and pioneer of the harm reduction, relapse prevention, and mindfulness-based therapies – whose innovative ideas and research have changed the way we view and treat addiction.

Mindfulness-Related Treatments and Addiction Recovery

Edited by
Marianne T. Marcus and Aleksandra Zgierska

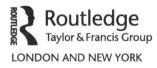

Routledge
Taylor & Francis Group

LONDON AND NEW YORK

First published 2012
by Routledge
2 Park Square, Milton Park, Abingdon, Oxon, OX14 4RN

Simultaneously published in the USA and Canada
by Routledge
711 Third Avenue, New York, NY 10017

First issued in paperback 2017

Routledge is an imprint of the Taylor & Francis Group, an informa business

British Library Cataloguing in Publication Data
A catalogue record for this book is available from the British Library

Typeset in Times New Roman
by Taylor & Francis Books

Publisher's Note
The publisher would like to make readers aware that the chapters in this book may be referred to as articles as they are identical to the articles published in the special issue. The publisher accepts responsibility for any inconsistencies that may have arisen in the course of preparing this volume for print.

ISBN 13: 978-1-138-11728-0 (pbk)
ISBN 13: 978-0-415-69689-0 (hbk)

Contents

CONTENTS

INTRODUCTION

Mindfulness-Based Therapies for Substance Use Disorders: Part 1

The link between stress and addiction is well known. Stress increases the likelihood of alcohol and drug use, and can precipitate relapses following treatment (1). Clinicians and researchers recognize the critical need to incorporate stress management techniques into inpatient and outpatient treatment. The goal is to assist clients to replace substance use with healthy coping skills when confronted with the inevitable stressors that threaten sobriety. Improved treatment retention and relapse prevention are desired outcomes of the challenging search for evidenced-based programs for recovering addicts.

This thematic issue of *Substance Abuse* is devoted to an emerging, promising area of research, mindfulness meditation as a therapy for addictive disorders. Conceptual framework and findings from pilot-level research combined with anecdotal evidence from clinical practice support the use of this innovative therapy for a broad spectrum of substance use disorders and mental health problems in general. If effective, mindfulness meditation–based interventions could help improve treatment outcomes in addictive disorders.

Mindfulness meditation, originally derived from Buddhist *Vipassana* meditation, is the cornerstone of the Mindfulness-Based Stress Reduction (MBSR) program developed by Kabat-Zinn in 1979 to teach patients with chronic physical and mental health problems how to improve their lives. MBSR is now used as an adjunctive treatment for a wide range of disorders and is increasingly finding its way into

the treatment of addiction. Kabat-Zinn defines mindfulness as "paying attention in a particular way: on purpose, in the present moment, and nonjudgmentally" (2). Mindfulness encourages awareness and acceptance of thoughts, feelings, and bodily sensations as they arise, and recognition of their impermanence. Mindfulness practitioners are taught to *acknowledge and accept* their experiences rather than to modify or suppress them. This change in one's relationship to present-moment experience has been described as "reperceiving" (3) or "attentional control" (4), and may facilitate more mindful behavioral responses. The set of skills associated with mindfulness can be taught independent of religious or cultural background, and in a variety of forms of interventions (5). In addition to MBSR, mindfulness-based interventions, used in a context of addictive disorders, include Mindfulness-Based Cognitive Therapy (MBCT) (6), Dialectical Behavior Therapy (DBT) (7), and Acceptance and Commitment Therapy (ACT) (8). Recent modifications of these approaches, developed specifically for substance abusing populations, include Mindfulness-Based Relapse Prevention (MBRP) (9) and Mindfulness-Based Therapeutic Community (MBTC) treatment (10).

The potential utility of mindfulness-based interventions for individuals in recovery from addictive disorders is particularly compelling. As an example, experiential avoidance, or an individual's unwillingness to remain in contact with unpleasant thoughts and experiences, has been implicated in substance abuse (11). Two studies showed that mindfulness meditation limits experiential avoidance by promoting nonjudgmental acceptance of moment-to-moment thoughts (12) and by interrupting the tendency to respond using maladaptive behaviors such as substance use (3). Craving, too, may be ameliorated by mindfulness practice as one learns not to react automatically but respond with awareness (13).

Although mindfulness meditation has been used in clinical settings as an adjunctive therapy for substance abuse for a long time, there has been a relative paucity of research in this field. When we "placed a call" for papers focused on mindfulness-based interventions targeting substance abuse, we were surprised by many submissions from multiple authors from a variety of clinical research settings around the world. Although this high turnout has exceeded our expectations, it highlights a growing interest in this clinical and research area. For this Special Issue of *Substance Abuse*, we accepted 10 excellent papers. Half of these articles is assembled in this issue, and the remaining 5 will be published in a subsequent issue of *Substance Abuse*.

The first paper by Zgierska and colleagues, "Mindfulness Meditation for Substance Use Disorders: A Systematic Review," is an extensive assessment of the clinical trial evidence of the effects of mindfulness-based therapies on addictive disorders. The authors found that although preliminary evidence suggests that mindfulness-based interventions are efficacious, the data are inconclusive; they also provided useful directions for further research to assist scholars in advancing the field.

Bowen and colleagues contributed "Mindfulness-Based Relapse Prevention for Substance Use Disorders: A Pilot Efficacy Trial," a study of MBRP for individuals who had recently completed intensive inpatient or outpatient addiction treatment. They report that MBRP participants, compared to those who received usual treatment only, experienced greater decreases in craving, and greater increases in acceptance and acting with awareness.

In "Mindfulness Training and Stress Reactivity in Substance Abuse: Results from a Random-

ized, Controlled Stage 1 Pilot Study," Brewer and colleagues compared a manualized version of mindfulness training to cognitive behavior therapy (CBT) for individuals in community-based outpatient addiction treatment. This study, which combined a laboratory-based behavioral experiment with psychological and physiological measures, suggested a reduction in stress-related indices in the mindfulness group compared to the CBT group.

The last two papers are derived from the same main study and report findings of cross-sectional analyses of baseline (precessation) data of 158 smokers enrolled in a smoking cessation trial comparing effects of MBSR to a standard of care treatment. Vidrine and colleagues examined the "Associations of Mindfulness with Nicotine Dependence, Withdrawal and Agency," and found that mindfulness was negatively associated with the level of nicotine dependence and "anticipatory" withdrawal severity, and positively associated with a sense of agency related to cessation. In the same sample of individuals, Waters and colleagues evaluated "Associations Between Mindfulness and Implicit Cognition and Self-Reported Affect" and noted that degree of mindfulness was negatively associated with severity of self-reported negative affect, perceived stress and depressive symptoms, and positively associated with positive affect level.

Combined, these studies offer an intriguing glimpse into the continuing quest for appropriate strategies to reduce stress and improve treatment outcomes in an especially vulnerable population, individuals with substance use disorders. A forthcoming issue of *Substance Abuse* will continue this theme with articles that look at effects of other mindfulness-based interventions in a range of substance-abusing client populations. The papers in the second issue will illustrate the ways in which mindfulness practice has been combined with other behavioral treatments and/or adapted to meet the needs of specific client populations (14–18).

REFERENCES

1. Sinha R. The role of stress in addiction relapse. *Curr Psychiatry Rep.* 2007;9:388–395.

2. Kabat-Zinn J. *Wherever You Go There You Are.* New York: Hyperion; 1994:4.

3. Shapiro SL, Carlson LE, Astin JA, Freedman B. Mechanisms of mindfulness. *J Clin Psychol.* 2006;62:373–386.

4. Teasdale JD, Segal Z, Williams JMG. How does cognitive therapy prevent depressive relapse and why should control (mindfulness) training help? *Behav Res Ther.* 1995;33:25–39.

5. Baer RA, Krietemeyer J. Overview of mindfulness- and acceptance-based treatment approaches. In: Baer RA, ed. *Mindfulness-Based Treatment Approaches: Clinician's Guide to Evidence Base and Applications.* New York: Academic Press; 2006:3–27.

6. Segal Z, Williams JMG, Teasdale JD. *Mindfulness-Based Cognitive Therapy for Depression: A New Approach to Preventing Relapse.* New York: Guilford; 2002.

7. Linehan MM. *Cognitive-Behavioral Treatment of Borderline Personality Disorder.* New York: Guilford Press; 1993.

8. Hayes SC. Acceptance, mindfulness, and science. *Clin Psychol Sci Pract.* 2002;9:101–106.

9. Witkiewitz K, Marlatt GA, Walker D. Mindfulness-based relapse prevention for alcohol and substance use disorders. *J Cogn Psychother.* 2005;19:211–228.

10. Marcus MT, Schmitz J, Moeller G, Liehr P, Cron SG, Swank P, Bankston S, Carroll D, Granmayeh LK. Mindfulness-based stress reduction in therapeutic community treatment: a stage 1 trial. *J Alcohol Drug Abuse.* 2009;35:103–108.

11. Hayes SC, Strosahl K, Wilson KG, Bissett RT, Pistorello J, Taormino D, Polusny MA, Dykstra TA, Batten SV, Began J, Stewart SH, Zvolensky MJ, Eifert GH, Bond FW, Forsyth JP, Karekla M, Mccurry SM. Measuring experiential avoidance: a preliminary test of a working model. *Psychol Rec.* 2004;54:553–578.

12. Simpson TL, Kaysen D, Bowen S, MacPherson LM, Chawla N, Blume A, Marlatt GA, Larimer ME. PTSD symptoms, substance abuse, and vipassana meditation among incarcerated individuals. *J Trauma Stress.* 2007;20:239–249.

13. Hsu SH, Grow J, Marlatt GA. Mindfulness and addiction. *Recent Dev Alcohol.* 2008;18:229–250.

14. Liehr P, Marcus MT, Carroll D, Granmayeh LK, Cron SG, Pennebaker JW. Linguistic analysis to assess the effect of a mindfulness intervention on self-change for adults in substance use recovery. *Subst Abuse.* In press.

15. Britton WB, Bootzin RR, Cousins JC, Hasler BP, Peck T, Shapiro SL. The contribution of mindfulness practice to a multicomponent behavioral sleep intervention following substance abuse treatment in adolescents: a treatment-development study. *Subst Abuse.* In press.

16. Smout MF, Longo M, Harrison S, Minniti R, Wickes W, White JM. Psychosocial treatment for methamphetamine use disorders: a preliminary randomized controlled trial of cognitive behavior therapy and acceptance and commitment therapy. *Subst Abuse.* In press.

17. Vieten C, Astin JA, Buscemi R, Galloway GP. Development of an acceptance-based coping intervention for alcohol dependence relapse prevention. *Subst Abuse.* In press.

18. Amaro H, Cielo Magno-Gatmaytan C, Meléndez M, Cortés DE, Arevalo S, Margolin A. Addiction treatment intervention: an uncontrolled prospective pilot study of spiritual self-schema therapy with Latina women. *Subst Abuse.* In press.

Marianne T. Marcus, EdD, RN, FAAN
Center for Substance Abuse Education,
Prevention, and Research
University of Texas Health Science
Center-Houston School of Nursing
Houston, TX

Aleksandra Zgierska, MD, PhD
Department of Family Medicine
University of Wisconsin, School of Medicine
and Public Health, Madison, WI

Mindfulness Meditation for Substance Use Disorders:
A Systematic Review

Aleksandra Zgierska, MD, PhD
David Rabago, MD
Neharika Chawla, MS
Kenneth Kushner, PhD
Robert Koehler, MLS
Alan Marlatt, PhD

ABSTRACT. Relapse is common in substance use disorders (SUDs), even among treated individuals. The goal of this article was to systematically review the existing evidence on mindfulness meditation-based interventions (MM) for SUDs. The comprehensive search for and review of literature found over 2000 abstracts and resulted in 25 eligible manuscripts (22 published, 3 unpublished: 8 randomized controlled trials, 7 controlled nonrandomized, 6 noncontrolled prospective, and 2 qualitative studies, and 1 case report). When appropriate, methodological quality, absolute risk reduction, number needed to treat, and effect size were assessed. Overall, although preliminary evidence suggests MM efficacy and safety, conclusive data for MM as a treatment of SUDs are lacking. Significant methodological limitations exist in most studies. Further, it is unclear which persons with SUDs might benefit most from MM. Future trials must be of sufficient sample size to answer a specific clinical question and should target both assessment of effect size and mechanisms of action.

INTRODUCTION

According to the United Nations Office on Drugs and Crime (1), approximately 200 million people worldwide are current drug users. In the United States, an estimated 22.6 million were diagnosed with substance dependence or abuse in 2006 (2). The cost of drug abuse worldwide, in terms of crime, loss of work, and health care costs, was estimated at 180.9 billion USD in 2002 (3). The human suffering related to substance use disorders is immeasurable.

Substance use disorders (SUDs) have been described as "chronic relapsing conditions," with rates of relapse exceeding 60% and being relatively consistent across substances of abuse (4–6). A range of treatments have been developed to target relapse. Among behavioral

Aleksandra Zgierska, David Rabago, and Kenneth Kushner are affiliated with the Department of Family Medicine, University of Wisconsin, School of Medicine and Public Health, Madison, Wisconsin, USA.

Neharika Chawla and Alan Marlatt are affiliated with the Addictive Behaviors Research Center, Department of Psychology, University of Washington, Seattle, Washington, USA.

Robert Koehler is affiliated with Meriter Hospital Library, Meriter Hospital, Madison, Wisconsin, USA.

This study was supported by grants from the National Institute on Alcohol Abuse and Alcoholism (5T32 AA014845—A.Z., and K23 AA017508—A.Z.).

interventions, cognitive behavioral therapy (CBT), including relapse prevention (7), has received considerable support. However, in spite of best "standard of care" therapy, relapse rates continue to be high, highlighting the need for development of new treatment modalities to better assist individuals in their recovery.

The theoretical framework for mindfulness meditation suggests that it may be a promising approach to treating addictive disorders (8,9). *Mindfulness* has been defined as the intentional, accepting, and nonjudgmental focus of one's attention on the emotions, thoughts, and sensations occurring in the present moment (10). Such a purposeful control of attention can be learned through training in techniques such as *meditation* (11). The "observe and accept" approach, characteristic of meditation, refers to being fully present and attentive to current experience but not being preoccupied by it. Thus, meditation can become a mental position for being able to separate a given experience from an associated emotion (12), and can facilitate a skillful or *mindful* response to a given situation (8). Meditation is often contrasted with everyday, habitual mental functioning or being on "autopilot." As such, meditation may be a valuable technique for SUD-affected persons, whose condition is often associated with unwanted thoughts, emotions, and sensations (e.g., craving), the tendency to be on "autopilot," and preoccupation with the "next fix," rather than "being in the present moment." Meditation may also be a component of maintaining lifestyle balance, with meditation-acquired skills complementing and enhancing CBT effects for SUDs (7,8,13,14).

Traditionally, meditative techniques have been taught and practiced through formal and informal meditation centers. More recently, meditation has also become a component of many therapeutic programs; in 1997, over 240 meditation programs were a part of U.S. health care systems (15), and the basics of meditation are taught in many U.S. medical schools. Mindfulness-Based Stress Reduction (MBSR) (10) is the most frequently cited method of mindfulness training in the medical context (16). Based on the MBSR model, other therapies combining both mindfulness and CBT elements have been developed, including the Mindfulness-Based Cognitive

Therapy (MBCT) for relapse related to recurrent depression (17) and Mindfulness-Based Relapse Prevention (MBRP) for relapse related to SUDs (9,18). Mindfulness is also a central part of Dialectical Behavior Therapy (DBT) for individuals with borderline personality disorder (19), Acceptance and Commitment Therapy (ACT) (20) for individuals with a variety of mental health problems, and Spiritual Self-Schema (3-S) therapy designed for clients with SUDs (21).

Although the use of mindfulness meditation as a therapy for SUDs is not new and has been associated with anecdotal clinical success (14), until recently there has been a paucity of research to support its empirical efficacy. The growing interest in complementary and alternative medicine (CAM), especially mind-body therapies (15,22), has brought a surge of interest in research evaluating the effects of meditation in a range of clinical contexts, including addictive problems. The current evidence on the clinical applications of mindfulness meditation for SUDs has not been rigorously reviewed.

The goal of this article was to systematically review and assess the existing evidence on the effects of mindfulness or mindfulness meditation–based therapies for addictive disorders. Although there are various forms of meditation, it is not known whether these approaches have similar effects on the problems or disorders under consideration. This review focused specifically on mindfulness meditation, and the term "meditation," as used in this review, refers exclusively to mindfulness meditation.

METHODS

Criteria for Selection of Studies

Inclusion criteria: (1) study intervention was mindfulness or mindfulness meditation based (MM); (2) used as a therapy for substance use, misuse or related disorders; (3) the study was longitudinal, with pre- and post-intervention assessments; and (4) it involved human subjects. *Exclusion criteria*: (1) lack of a sufficient description of the study intervention to determine if it was rooted in mindfulness; (2) non-English; and (3) only interim results of an unpublished

TABLE 1. Electronic Database Search Strategy

Step	Search strategy
1	Meditation [tw] or relaxation [tw] or mindfulness [tw] or "breathing technique" [tw] or "breathing exercises" [tw]
2	Smoking [tw] or tobacco [tw] or caffeine [tw] or "substance-related disorder" [tw] or "drug abuse" [tw] or addiction [tw] or "drug dependence" [tw] or "drug habituation" [tw] or "drug usage" [tw] or "substance abuse" [tw] or "substance dependence" [tw] or "substance use" [tw] or alcohol [tw] or alcoholism [tw] or "street drugs" [tw] or cocaine [tw] or marijuana [tw] or marihuana [tw] or opioid [tw] or heroin [tw] or morphine [tw] or stimulant [tw] or ecstasy [tw] or nicotine [tw]
3	1 and 2

study were available. We anticipated that the number of eligible studies would be limited; therefore, we did not exclude studies based on design (experimental versus nonexperimental), methodological quality, or specific intervention protocol. Both published and unpublished reports were eligible for inclusion.

Search Strategy

The research librarian (R.K.) worked closely with the coauthors (A.Z., K.K.) to refine search strategies. Comprehensive searches (Table 1) were conducted through March 9, 2008, of the following electronic databases: Cochrane Database of Systematic Reviews (since 1995), EMBASE (since 1993), PubMed (including PreMed and Old Med, since 1950), PsycINFO (since 1967), CINAHL (since 1982), and Allied and Complementary Medicine (since 1985). The National Institutes of Health (NIH) CRISP electronic database of relevant institutes (National Institute on Alcohol Abuse and Alcoholism, National Institute on Drug Abuse, National Institute of Mental Health, National Center for Complementary and Alternative Medicine) was searched from 1995 to March 9, 2008, with keywords "meditation" OR "mindfulness." The Scientific Research on The Transcendental Meditation Program: Collected Papers (Volumes 1 to 4) were hand-searched. The reference lists of relevant articles were reviewed to identify potentially eligible studies. E-mail or phone

contact was attempted with relevant author(s) or Principle Investigator(s) of included articles or abstracts when additional information was needed.

Identification of Eligible Studies

The titles and abstracts of all identified studies were screened (R.K. and A.Z., "initial screening"). Studies that clearly described using only Transcendental Meditation, Progressive Muscle Relaxation, Biofeedback, or Autogenic Training as their interventions were excluded. The full-text of studies describing the use of meditation, mindfulness, relaxation, yoga, breath practices, or other techniques that were compatible or potentially compatible with mindfulness meditation (as the primary or comparison interventions) were then reviewed (A.Z., "secondary screening"). Practices that were included as compatible with MM are described in the following section. The secondary screening resulted in an exclusion of ineligible articles (A.Z.); articles that were considered potentially eligible were then additionally reviewed ("tertiary screening") by 3 independent reviewers (N.C., G.A.M., K.K.), experts in psychology, meditation, and relapse prevention for SUDs.

Data Extraction and Study Assessments

Data from all eligible articles were extracted, and the methodological quality of controlled and prospective case series studies was assessed for internal validity by 2 unblinded reviewers (A.Z., D.R.). We used an adapted version of a scoring instrument suited for studies using behavioral interventions and developed for the systematic review of alcohol treatment trials (23). This instrument (Table 2) was adapted for use in SUDs with input from Dr. William Miller, codeveloper of the original scale (personal communication, March–April, 2008).

Using this instrument, the studies were assigned the following subscores (Table 3): (a) Population Severity Rating (PSR); (b) Methodological Quality Score (MQS); (c) Clinical Benefit Score (CBS; called the Outcome Logic Score in the original scale (23)); and (d) Cumulative Evidence Score (CES), where CES = CBS ×

TABLE 2. Scoring* of the Prospective Studies (Range of Points): Population Severity Rating (PSR), Clinical Benefit Score (CBS), Methodological Quality Score (MQS), and Cumulative Evidence Score (CES)

PSR (range: 0–4)	0 = insufficient information; 1 = nonclinical sample, mild or no problems; 2 = nonclinical sample of nicotine dependent smokers; or drug users or problem drinkers who did not seek treatment and did not have severe problems or dependence; 3 = clinical sample of drug users or problem drinkers who sought treatment for substance use related problems, but who did not have dependence; 4 = severely impaired clinical population in treatment for drug or alcohol dependence.
CBS (range: −2 to +2)	+2 = <u>controlled trials:</u> MM was significantly better than 'no Tx' (MM > 0); or MM combined with other Tx was significantly better than that Tx alone (MM+A > A); <u>noncontrolled trials:</u> significant improvement on primary outcome post- vs. pre-intervention.
	+1 = <u>controlled trials:</u> MM was significantly better than an alternative Tx (including SOC), or better than a briefer form of the same MM therapy, without control (MM > A); <u>noncontrolled trials:</u> significant improvement post- vs. pre-intervention on secondary outcome only.
	−1 = <u>controlled trials:</u> MM outcomes were comparable to those of an alternative Tx (MM = A) or MM combined with other Tx (MM = MM+A), or briefer form of the same MM therapy, or mixed differences among active Tx arms, without control; <u>noncontrolled trials:</u> no significant change in any outcomes post- vs. pre-intervention.
	−2 = <u>controlled trials:</u> MM was worse than a comparable other Tx of similar intensity without control (MM < A), or not better than a briefer dissimilar Tx without control, or MM combined with other Tx produced worse results than other Tx alone (MM+A < A), or MM is not better than no-Tx (MM ≤ 0); <u>noncontrolled trials:</u> no improvement, but presence of worsening in the outcomes post- vs. pre-intervention.
MQS (range: 0–17) Noncontrolled trials: maximum score = 12	• Group allocation: 4 = randomization, 3 = within-S counterbalanced, 2 = case control/matching, 1 = quasiexperimental design, arbitrary assignment, sequential, cohorts; 0 = violated randomization or nonequivalent groups (or noncontrolled trial).
	• Quality control: 1 = Tx standardized by manual, specific training, content coding, etc.; 0 = no standardization is specified.
	• Follow-up rate (at any follow-up point): 2 = 85–100%; 1 = 70–84.9%; 0 = fewer than 70%, or longest follow-up <3 months.
	• Follow-up length: 2 = at least 12 months; 1 = 6–11 months; 0 = less than 6 months, or unspecified.
	• Contact: 1 = personal for ≥70% of completed cases; 0 = nonpersonal or unspecified, or in <70% of cases.
	• Collateral interviews: 1 = present in >50% of cases; 0 = present in ≤50% of cases, or unspecified.
	• Objective verification: 1 = present in >50% of cases (records, biomarkers); 0 = absent in ≤ 50% of cases, or unspecified.
	• Attrition: 2 = both Tx drop-outs AND cases lost to follow-up are enumerated, AND are considered in outcome; 1 = meets "considered" criteria for either drop-outs OR cases lost to follow-up, but not both; 0 = dropped and lost cases are not considered in outcome (e.g., all noncompleters are excluded from outcome analyses).
	• Independent: 1 = assessors are independent and blind to group; 0 = follow-up nonblind, unspecified (or noncontrolled trial).
	• Analyses: 1 = acceptable analyses of group differences (or pre-post analyses for noncontrolled trials); 0 = no statistical analysis, inappropriate, or unspecified.
	• Multisite: 1 = parallel replications at ≥2 sites, separate research teams; 0 = single site or sites offering different Tx.
CES	CES score = CBS × MQS (range for an individual study: −34 to +34) Negative (−) CES indicates studies showing a comparable or worse Tx outcome, positive (+) CES indicates studies showing a significant benefit of the MM therapy, compared to a comparison group in controlled trials, or baseline in uncontrolled trials.

Note. MM = mindfulness or mindfulness meditation–based intervention; SOC = standard of care; Tx = treatment.
*Adapted with permission from William Miller (personal communication, 2008) (23).

MQS. (e) The Overall CES was also calculated for subgroups of studies (e.g., randomized controlled trials [RCTs]), as a sum of CES of individual studies.

When possible, absolute risk reduction (ARR), number needed to treat (NNT), and effect size (ES) were calculated by the authors (A.Z., D.R.) for the main substance use–related outcomes. The following formulas were used: (a) ARR = absolute difference in outcome rates between the control and treatment groups; (b) NTT = 1/ARR; and (c) ES, Cohen's d, was either converted from correlations (where $r = .37$ corresponded to $d = .8$, $r = .24$ corresponded to $d = .5$, and $r = .1$ corresponded to $d = .2$) or calculated from the mean values (M) and standard deviations (SDs); Cohen's d for controlled trials was calculated as

$$d = [M1 - M2]/SD_{pooled}, \qquad (1)$$

where M1, M2 were the means in the 2 groups, and $SD_{pooled} = \sqrt{[(SD1^2 + SD2^2)/2]}$. Cohen's d for uncontrolled pre-post trials was calculated as

$$d = [\text{mean of the pre} - \text{post difference}]/$$
$$[\text{SD of this mean}]). \qquad (2)$$

In cases where it was not possible to use Equation 2, then Equation 1 was used.

RESULTS

Literature Search Results (Figure 1)

The search identified 1095 abstracts of published articles. After removing 595 duplicates (R.K.), 500 abstracts were reviewed (A.Z., initial screening). Of those, 276 were excluded. The full-texts of 224 articles were then reviewed

FIGURE 1. Results of the literature search. (DB, database)

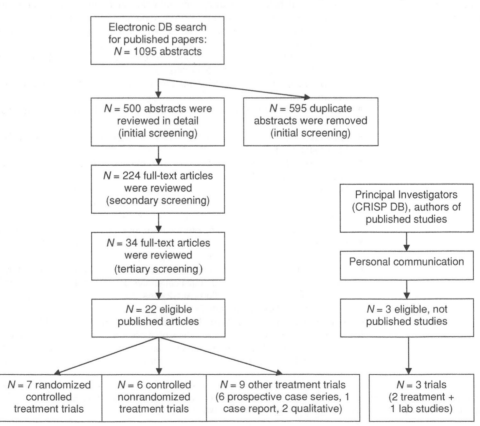

(A.Z., secondary screening), and 34 articles were submitted for a tertiary screening. Twelve of the 34 articles (24–35) did not meet the eligibility criteria and were excluded. Of the excluded studies, two deserve an additional comment (24,34). Both studies used the body scan technique as a study intervention. Although the body scan was derived from a mindfulness meditation–based program, in isolation, this technique did not meet the criteria for mindfulness or mindfulness meditation because MM-based body scan involves not only instructions on paying attention to the various parts of the body, but also encourages focused awareness, without attempt to change or manipulate body sensations, thus promoting nonjudgmental and compassionate acceptance of whatever is occurring in the body at any given moment.

The 22 published articles included 7 RCTs (36–42), 6 controlled nonrandomized trials (43–48), 6 prospective case series (49–53), 1 case report (54), and 2 qualitative studies (55,56). Seventeen of these reports were based on separate clinical trials and 5 on secondary database analyses (45,48,52,55,57). The CRISP database search found 324 "hits," resulting in 9 additional relevant abstracts. Through personal communication, 2 ready-for-submission, but unpublished articles (58,59) and 1 PhD dissertation (60) were additionally identified as eligible, resulting in a total of 25 included studies. Of note, since completion of this review, results of one of the "unpublished studies" (58) have been published (61).

The heterogeneity of the included studies and interrater agreement on methodological quality scoring were not formally assessed. The wide variety of conditions treated, treatment protocols, and outcome measures used was apparent on inspection, and made the pooling of data impossible. Disagreements between the reviewers were resolved by consensus.

Methods of the Included Published Studies (Tables 3 to 5)

Studied Population

Three studies focused on adolescents (49,52,57), whereas the remaining 19 studies evaluated adults. Of the 22 studies, 12 evaluated severely impaired subjects (Population Severity Rating [PSR] 4/4), treated for alcohol and/or drug dependence in residential (36,46,51,56), or outpatient settings (37,40,41,47,53,55,62), 3 described a clinical sample of adolescents with SUDs (PSR 3/4) (49,52,57), 3 included a nonclinical sample of substance-using prisoners (PSR 2/4) (44,45,48), and 4 were based on community-recruited adults (PSR 2/4) with tobacco (38,43,50) or marijuana (54) dependence.

MM Intervention

The MM interventions used in the included studies were based on 5 main models:

Vipassana meditation (http://www.dhamma. org). This is a form of MM that is deeply rooted in the Buddhist tradition. Most contemporary forms of MM derive from traditional Vipassana meditation. Typical Vipassana courses are group-based, last 10 consecutive days, are conducted in silence, and involve meditating for 10 to 11 hours per day. They are available at no charge and follow a similar curriculum worldwide.

Three articles (44,45,48), based on one study (44), described the effects of a traditional Vipassana training led by a traditionally trained teacher, in a prison settings. The intervention was standardized (followed a traditional Vipassana format), but its delivery was not monitored.

Mindfulness-Based Stress Reduction (MBSR). Originally developed for management of chronic pain and stress-related disorders (10), MBSR has been shown to be effective or potentially effective for many mental health and medical conditions (16). MBSR is the most frequently cited method of meditation training in the medical context (16), and has a published curriculum (10). The usual MBSR course consists of 8 weekly, therapist-led group sessions (2 to 2.5 hours per session), one full-day retreat (7 to 8 hours), and daily home assignments. The MBSR curriculum served as a model for the manualized Mindfulness-Based Cognitive Therapy (MBCT) (17) that combines meditation (10) and traditional cognitive therapy strategies (63) to prevent relapse in recurrent depression. MBCT has been shown to reduce the rate of depressive

TABLE 3. Summary of the Cumulative Evidence Scores of the Published Included Studies

Studies	Number of studies	Methodological Quality Score (MQS) (mean/17)	Population Severity Score, PSS (mean/4)	Cumulative Evidence Score (CES) (sum of scores of the individual studies)	% positive (% studies with +CES)
Total	15*	8.0	3.3	ITT: +10 (6 studies) PP: +143 (13 studies)	ITT: 50% PP: 85%
By design					
RCTs	7	11.3 (range: 8–14)	3.7	ITT: +2 (4 studies) PP: +93 (6 studies)	ITT: 50% PP: 83%
Controlled, nonrandomized	4*	6.8 (range: 6–8)	3	ITT: −8 (1 study) PP: +16 (3 studies)	ITT: 0% PP: 67%
Case series	4	5.8 (range: 4–8)	3.25	ITT: +16 (1 study) PP: +34 (4 studies)	ITT: 100% PP: 100%
By MM intervention					
DBT	2 RCTs	13.5 (13, 14)	4	ITT: +27 (2 studies) PP: +13 (1 study)	ITT: 100% PP: 100%
ACT	2 RCTs	12.5 (12, 13)	3	ITT: −25 (2 studies) PP: +50 (2 studies)	ITT: 0% PP: 100%
3-S	3 (2 RCT, 1 controlled)	8.7 (range: 7–11)	4	ITT: — (0 studies) PP: +26 (3 studies)	ITT: — PP: 67%
MBSR-based	7* (1 RCT, 2 controlled, 4 case series)	6.4 (range: 4–8)	3.3	ITT: +8 (2 studies) PP: +42 (6 studies)	ITT: 50% PP: 83%
Vipassana	1 controlled	6	2	ITT: — (0 studies) PP: +12 (1 study)	ITT: — PP: 100%
By subject population					
SUDs, adults, outpatient settings	7 (5 RCTs, 1 controlled, 1 case series)	10.3 (range: 7–14)	4	ITT: +15 (3 studies) PP: +69 (6 studies)	ITT: 67% PP: 83%
SUDs, adults, tobacco dependence	3* (1 RCT, 1 controlled, 1 case series)	9 (6, 8, 13)	2	ITT: +3 (2 studies) PP: +42 (2 studies)	ITT: 50% PP: 100%
SUDs, adults, residential settings	3 (1 RCT, 1 controlled, 1 case series)	6.7 (4, 8, 8)	4	ITT: −8 (1 study) PP: +12 (3 studies)	ITT: 0% PP: 67%
Substance use, adults, jail	1 controlled	6	2	ITT: — (0 studies) PP: +12 (1 study)	ITT: — PP: 100%
Substance use, adolescents	1 case series	4	3	ITT: — (0 studies) PP: +8 (1 study)	ITT: — PP: 100%

Note. The studies are grouped by study design, type of mindfulness or mindfulness meditation intervention (MM), and subject population, sorted within groups by the mean Methodological Quality Score of the studies.
*One nonrandomized controlled study did not use statistical analysis to compare results.

relapse among persons with recurrent depression (64,65) and may be efficacious for symptom reduction in "active" depression (66) and anxiety disorders as well (67). Using the MBCT model in turn, a manualized Mindfulness-Based Relapse Prevention (MBRP) program has been developed for outpatient clients with SUDs (9, 18). The elements of cognitive therapy in MBRP are based on relapse prevention cognitive therapy strategies (7) that have demonstrated efficacy for SUDs (68). Evaluation of the MBRP program for SUDs is currently ongoing (69).

Ten articles (36,43,46,49–53,56,57), based on 8 separate studies (36,43,46,49–51,53,56), reported use of the MBSR-based intervention. Only one study did not report modifications to the MBSR curriculum (43); the other studies implemented modified MBSR programs, tailored to the targeted population. The modifications were reported as "minor" in 3 studies (46,50,51)—in these studies, the intervention, delivered by trained MBSR teachers, was labeled as "MBSR" and scored as "manualized." Two studies (4 reports: 36,49,52,57) used

TABLE 4. Published RCTs of Mindfulness or Mindfulness Meditation–Based Interventions (MM) Used for the Treatment of Substance Use, Misuse, or Disorders

Feature	Study 1. Alterman et al. 2004 (36)	Study 2. Avants et al. 2005 (37)	Study 3. Margolin et al. 2006 (42)	Study 4. Hayes et al. 2004 (39)	Study 5. Gifford et al. 2004 (38)	Study 6. Linehan et al. 1999 (41)	Study 7. Linehan et al. 2002 (40)
Subjects	31 (17 F); mean age 36.5 yrs	29 (17 F); mean age 41.7 (28–51 yrs)	72 (47 F); mean age ~ 41 (21–56 yrs)	124 (63 F); mean age 42.2 (23–64 yrs); anxiety and/or mood disorders ~ 42%	76 (45 F); mean age 43 (19–71 yrs)	28 F; mean age 30.4 (18–45 yrs); 50% depression, 38% PTSD	23 F; mean age 36.1 (18–45 yrs); anxiety and/or mood disorders 40–50%; past suicide or self-injury attempt 65%
Addictive disorder	PSR 4; SUDs, recovery house residents; alcohol + drugs 68%.	PSR 4; opiate- & cocaine-dependent methadone maintenance outpatients.	PSR 4; opiate-dependent methadone maintenance outpatients.	PSR 4; poly-SUDs; Opiate-dependent methadone maintenance outpatients.	PSR 2; tobacco-dependent community-recruited adults, with at least one past-year quit attempt; on average, smoked 21.4 cig/day.	PSR 4; BPD + SUDs; recruited from the clinic patients; 74% poly-SUDs, 58% cocaine, 52% alcohol.	PSR 4; BPD + opiate dependence; recruited from variety of outpatient settings; 52% cocaine, 26% alcohol, 13% sedative dependent.
MM group & MM intervention	N = 18; MBSR-based, 8 wks: therapist-led group sessions (120 min/wk) & one retreat (7 hrs) + 30–45-min meditation group meetings (4 times/wk).	N = 11; 3-S (individual), 8 wks: therapist-led individual sessions (60 min/wk).	N = 38; 3-S (2 groups), 8 wks: one educational session (60 min), AND • N = 20; therapist-led individual sessions (60 min/wk), OR • N = 18; therapist-led individual (60 min/wk) & group (60 min/wk) sessions.	N = 42; ACT, 16 wks: therapist-led 32 individual (60-min) & 16 group (90-min) sessions.	N = 33; ACT, 7 wks: therapist-led 7 individual (50 min/wk) & 7 group (90 min/wk) sessions.	N = 12; DBT for SUDs, 52 wks: therapist-led individual (60 min/wk) & group (120 min/wk) sessions + skills coaching calls + optional 39-wk methadone or methylphenidate Tx for opiate or stimulant dependence.	N = 11; DBT for SUDs, 52 wks: therapist-led individual (40–90 min/wk) & group (150 min/wk) sessions + optional individual coaching (30 min/wk) + diary cards.

(Continued on next page)

TABLE 4. (Continued)

Feature	Study 1. Alterman et al. 2004 (36)	Study 2. Avants et al. 2005 (37)	Study 3. Margolin et al. 2006 (42)	Study 4. Hayes et al. 2004 (39)	Study 5. Gifford et al. 2004 (38)	Study 6. Linehan et al. 1999 (41)	Study 7. Linehan et al. 2002 (40)
Comparison group (CG)	$N = 13$, SOC only.	$N = 18$; 3-S (individual & group); 8 wks: therapist-led individual (60 min/wk) & group (60 min/wk) sessions.	$N = 34$; 'waitlist' SOC only.	• $N = 44$; ITSF, 16 wks: 32 individual (60 min) therapist or AA sponsor-led, +16 group (90-min) therapist-led sessions. • $N = 38$; SOC only.	$N = 43$; NRT + medical Tx (physician-led): one 90-min group education session; then weekly clinic visits (physician visit as needed).	$N = 16$; SOC only (subjects were referred to other clinics for SOC).	$N = 12$; CVT + 12-Step, 52 wks: individual (40–90 min/wk) + NA group (120 min/wk) + optional 12-Step meetings.
Ancillary treatment (all groups)	SOC	One 60-min individual HIV educational session + SOC	SOC	SOC	None	None	ORLAAM (52 wks), physician-led medical Tx; weekly UTox; case management; PTSD Tx, crisis intervention, 12-Step.
Follow-up:	0, 8, 22 wks	0, 8 wks	0, 8 wks	0, 8, 16, 42 wks	0, 7, 26, 52 wks	0, 16, 32, 52, 68 wks	0, 16, 32, 52, 68 wks
Retention (at the end of follow-up):	• MM 83%; • CG 77%	• MM (Individual) 64%; • MM (individual + group) 89%	• MM 82%; • CG 88%	• MM 43%; • ITSF 57%; • CG 68% (differential retention: $P < .07$).	• MM 61%; • CG 81% (differential retention: $P = .07$)	• MM 58%; • CG 50%	• MM 82%; • CG
Outcome measures	Drug use (self-report, UTox); psychological health, problem level; meditation practice	Drug use (self-report, UTox); HIV risk behavior, spirituality (surveys, reaction time task); Tx experiences.	Drug use (HIV risk behavior survey, with "yes/no" question on injection drug use or unprotected sex; UTox), HIV prevention motivation; spirituality (surveys, reaction time task); Tx experiences.	Drug use (self-report, UTox); psychopathology; Tx satisfaction.	Tobacco use (self-report, exhaled CO); dependence, withdrawal symptoms, psychological health; Tx experience.	Drug use (self-report, UTox); prior Tx, parasuicide history, psychological health.	Drug use (self-report, UTox); parasuicide history, psychological health, Brief Symptom Inventory.

Substance use-related outcomes (per ITT & PP analyses, at the end of follow-up, unless stated otherwise)	ITT: N/A; PP: ● no differences between the groups (ES <.1); ● compared to baseline, both groups decreased substance use.	ITT: N/A; PP: ● no differences between the groups; ● compared to baseline, the groups (combined into one sample) decreased heroin and cocaine use ($P < .05$ [ES .5]) and HIV risk behavior ($P = .08$ [ES .4]); ● all but one subject reported positive 3-S effects on drug use, craving, motivation for abstinence and HIV prevention.	ITT: N/A; PP: ● compared to SOC controls, fewer 3-S subjects injected drugs and/or had unsafe sex (53% vs. 23%, $P < .05$ [ARR 30%, NNT 3.3]); ● receipt of 3-S therapy was an independent protective factor against engaging in these behaviors (OR 8.9, $P < .05$); ● 3-S attendance was correlated to HIV risk behaviors ($r = -.33$, $P < .05$; [ES .7]).	ITT: ● no significant differences between the ACT, ITSF and SOC groups (no details provided); PP: ● the ACT and ITSF groups, compared to SOC, had more 'clean' UTox for opiates (61%, 50%, 28%, $P < .05$ [ACT vs. SOC: ARR 33%, NNT 3.0; ACT vs. ITSF: ARR 11%, NNT 9.1]) and all drugs (50%, 38%, 12%, $P < .05$ [ACT vs. SOC: ARR 38%, NNT 2.6; ACT vs. ITSF: ARR 12%, NNT 8.3]); ● the ACT group tended to more accurately report drug use than the ITSF group ($P < .1$).	ITT: ● no significant difference in quit rate between the ACT and NRT groups (21% vs. 9%, $P > .05$ [ARR 12%, NNT 8.3]); PP: ● ACT had a better quit rate than the NRT group (35% vs. 15%, $P < .05$ [ARR 20%, NNT 5]); ● quit status was predicted by change in acceptance skills in the ACT group, and change in acceptance skills mediated effects of ACT on smoking status and predicted quit status in the ACT group ($P < .05$).	ITT: ● DBT group had a higher proportion of drug/alcohol abstinent days compared to SOC (94 vs. .58, $P < .05$, ES .59); PP: ● The above difference was significant (ES 1.0).	ITT: ● at 52 wks, DBT group reduced opiate use compared to CVT group ($P < .05$), however, this difference disappeared at 68 wks (positive UTox for opiates: 27% vs. 33%, $P > .05$ [ARR 5%; NNT 22]); ● during the 52-wk-long Tx, the DBT group was more accurate in substance use reporting than CVT group ($P < .05$). PP: N/A.
Other outcomes (per ITT & PP analyses, at the end of follow-up, unless stated otherwise)	ITT: N/A; PP: ● the Addiction Severity Index medical composite score improved in the MM, but not SOC group ($P < .05$, ES .195); ● 47% MM subjects continued meditating (4 hrs during the prior month).	ITT: N/A; PP: ● compared to baseline, 3-S subjects increased spiritual practices, and showed a cognitive shift from 'addict' to 'spiritual' self ($P < .05$); ● spirituality correlated to drug abstinence ($r = .6$, $P < .05$ [ES .4]) and to decrease in HIV risk behavior ($r = .67$, $P < .05$ [ES .45]).	ITT: N/A; PP: ● compared to SOC, 3-S group increased spiritual practices and motivation for HIV prevention, and showed a cognitive shift from 'addict' to 'spiritual qualities' ($P < .05$); ● all 3-S subjects reported meditating (mean 25.7 min/day) and planned continuing it.	ITT: N/A; PP: ● the ACT subjects endorsed better relationship with their providers than the NRT subjects ($P < .05$); ● Tx satisfaction ratings were comparable between the groups.	ITT: ● no differences between the groups in psychological health scores or Tx satisfaction ratings; ● compared to baseline, the groups improved on majority of psychological outcomes ($P < .05$). PP: Results as above.	(unclear whether ITT or PP was used): ● compared to SOC, the DBT group received more psychotherapy ($P < .05$), and improved the global adjustment and global social adjustment scores ($P < .05$).	ITT: ● no differences between the groups in psychopathology or jail time; ● compared to baseline, both groups improved the Brief Symptom Inventory scores and global adjustment ratings.

(Continued on next page)

TABLE 4. (Continued)

Feature	Study 1. Alterman et al. 2004 (36)	Study 2. Avants et al. 2005 (37)	Study 3. Margolin et al. 2006 (42)	Study 4. Hayes et al. 2004 (39)	Study 5. Gifford et al. 2004 (38)	Study 6. Linehan et al. 1999 (41)	Study 7. Linehan et al. 2002 (40)
Adverse effects	Not mentioned	Not mentioned	Not mentioned	Not mentioned	Not mentioned	Not mentioned	Not mentioned
MQS/17	8	8	11	12	13	13	14
CBS (ITT & PP analyses)	ITT: N/A PP: +2	ITT: N/A PP: −1	ITT: N/A PP: +2	ITT: −1 PP: +2	ITT: −1 PP: +2	ITT: +1 PP: +1	ITT: +1 PP: N/A
Comments	All subjects lived in the same recovery house.	The sample was randomized to individual or individual + group therapy; however, detailed results are reported as for pre-post one group.	After the initial randomization, the MM group was sub-randomized to individual ($N = 20$) or individual + group therapy ($N = 18$); in the final analysis, these subgroups were combined into one MM group.	3-Arm RCT, with 2 "active" interventions (MM and ITSF) that were "matched" by subject involvement and therapy format (but not therapist contact time).	None	Low Tx completion rate, especially in the SOC group (DBT 55%, SOC 19% per ITT).	Two interventions were "matched" by subject involvement and therapy format (but not therapist contact time). One subject was randomized incorrectly, removed before the study onset and not analyzed (resulting in $N = 23$). All drop-outs took place in the DBT group led by the only male therapist.

Note. In the Outcomes section, values presented in [square brackets] were calculated by the authors for this systematic review.
Values (presented in [square brackets]) calculated for the systematic review: ARR: absolute risk reduction; CBS: Clinical Benefit Score; CES: Cumulative Evidence Score; ES: effect size (Cohen's *d*); MQS: Methodological Quality Score; NNT: number needed to treat; PSS: Population Severity Score.
ACT: Acceptance Commitment Therapy; BPD: borderline personality disorder; CO: carbon monoxide; CVT: Comprehensive Validation Therapy; DBT: Dialectical Behavior Therapy; MM: mindfulness meditation; HIV: human immunodeficiency virus; ITSF: Intensive Twelve Step Facilitation; ITT: intention to treat analysis; MBSR: Mindfulness-Based Stress Reduction; min: minutes; mos: months; NRT: nicotine replacement therapy; ORLAAM: oral solution levomethadyl acetate, opiate agonist; PP: per protocol analysis; PTSD: post-traumatic stress disorder; 3-S: Spiritual Self Schema; SOC: "standard of care" therapy; SUDS: substance use disorders; TSF: Twelve Step Facilitation; Tx: treatment; UTox: urine toxicology test; wks: weeks; yrs: years.

TABLE 5. Published Controlled Nonrandomized Trials, Case Series, Case Report and Qualitative Studies of Mindfulness or Mindfulness Meditation–Based Interventions (MM) Used for the Treatment of Substance Use, Misuse, or Disorders: Methods and Results

Study	Indication	Subjects	Intervention	Outcome measures	Results	Methodological quality/comments
Controlled nonrandomized trials						
Study 1. Margolin et al. 2007 (47)	Substance use (as a part of HIV risk behavior assessment) in HIV-positive, opiate dependent, methadone maintenance outpatients.	38 (19 F); mean age 45.3 (33–57 yrs); PSR 4; 55% cocaine use disorder; 71% were prescribed an HIV Tx.	Per subject choice: • MM (N = 21), SOC + 3-S, 12 wks, therapist-led individual (60 min/wk) & group (60 min/wk) sessions; • CG (N = 17): SOC only.	• Collected at 0, 12 wks; • Substance use (self-report, UTox); • Drug- and sex-related HIV risk behaviors; • Impulsivity, spirituality; • Tx experiences.	• Retention: MM 67%, CG 65%; PP: • compared to CG, MM showed trend to decreased alcohol and drug use (P = .08 [ES .25]), improved impulsivity, spirituality and motivation for abstinence (P < .05); • 3-S attendance correlated to decreased substance use (ES .2), impulsivity, and increased influence of spirituality on abstinence and HIV prevention motivation (P < .05).	MQS: 7/17; CBS: N/A per ITT (+2 per PP); Meditation practice pattern, adverse effects and side effects were not reported.
Study 2a. Bowen et al. 2006 (44)	Substance use among prisoners of the minimum-security jail.	305 (63 F), mean age 37.5 (19–58 yrs); PSR 2; alcohol use 83%, tobacco use 83%, drug use 73% during 90 days prior to incarceration.	Per subject choice: • MM (N = 63): SOC + vipassana meditation (VM): 10 consecutive days: silent, gender-specific course, 8–10 hrs/day, led by a trained instructor; • CG (N = 242): SOC only.	• Collected at 0, 1 wk post-intervention, 3 & 6 mos post-release; • Substance use (self-report), related harms consequences; • Psychological health.	• Retention at 3 & 6 mos: MM 46% & 43%; CG 24% & 21%. PP: • At 3 mos, compared to CG, MM reduced (P < .05) alcohol [ES .6], cocaine [ES .35] and marijuana [ES .5] use, and alcohol-related harms [ES .35], improved psychiatric symptoms, drinking-related locus of control and optimism; the changes were related to the VM participation; • At 6 mos, recidivism rates (the only results reported for 6 mos) were low, and comparable between the groups.	MQS: 6/17; CBS: N/A per ITT (+2 per PP); Post-intervention meditation practice pattern, adverse effects and side effects were not reported.

(Continued on next page)

TABLE 5. (Continued)

Study	Indication	Subjects	Intervention	Outcome measures	Results	Methodological quality/comments
Study 2b. Bowen et al. 2007 (45) (secondary analysis of Study 2a).	Relationship between substance use & thought suppression; prisoners.	See Bowen et al. 2006 (44) $N = 81$ (for the main analysis of 0–3-month outcomes)	See Bowen et al. 2006 (44)	See Bowen et al. 2006 (44)	PP: • At 3 mos, compared to CG, MM decreased thought avoidance ($P < .05$); this change partially mediated the relationship between the VM participation, and alcohol use and related harms.	See Bowen et al. 2006 (44)
Study 2c. Simpson et al. 2007 (48) (secondary analysis of Study 2a).	Relationship between substance use & PTSD severity; prisoners	See Bowen et al. 2006 (44) $N = 88$: 29 MM and 59 CG (for the main analysis of 0–3-month outcomes)	See Bowen et al. 2006 (44)	See Bowen et al. 2006 (44)	PP: • No differences in the PTSD symptom severity between the MM and CG groups; VM participation and baseline substance use, but not PTSD severity, predicted alcohol and drug use at 3 mos; baseline PTSD severity predicted drinking related harms and psychological distress at 3 mos; PTSD subjects tolerated the VM course well;	See Bowen et al. 2006 (44)
Study 3. Altner 2002 (43)	Smoking cessation among tobacco-dependent hospital employees	114 (71 F), mean age ~ 38.5 (20–65 yrs); PSR 2	Per subject choice: • MM ($N = 49$): NRT + MBSR, 8 wks: therapist-led (2.5 hr/wk) group sessions; • CG ($N = 65$): NRT only.	• Collected at 0, 1.5, 3, 6, 15 mos (quit date likely at '0'); • % subjects who stopped, reduced or did not reduce smoking (self-report, exhaled CO); • Tx experiences among meditators ($N = 23$, qualitative) at 3 mos.	• Retention: MM 100%; CG 97%. Descriptive statistics: MM vs. CG subjects reported quit rate of 32.6% vs. 24.6% [ARR 8%, NNT 12.5], reduced smoking by 42.3% vs. 26.2%, continued smoking by 22.4% vs. 46.2%; • Qualitative data: meditators reported positive opinions on the MBSR therapy and its usefulness for coping.	MQS: 6/17; CBS: N/A Since no statistical assessment of the significance of in-between group differences or pre-post changes was provided; only descriptive statistics were used. Exhaled CO results were not reported.

Study	Aim	Sample	Design/Intervention	Measures	Results	Quality
Study 4. Marcus et al. 2001 (46)	Psychological health in alcohol or drug-dependent patients of therapeutic community	36 (2 F), mean age ~ 34 years; PSR 4	Per subject choice: • MM ($N = 18$): SOC + MBSR, 8 wks, therapist-led (2.5 hrs/wk) group sessions; • CG ($N = 18$): SOC only.	• Collected at 0, 8 wks; • Psychopathology (SCL-90R), coping styles.	• Retention: MM & CG 100%; ITT = PP: • Compared to CG, MM group tended to report a more self-controlling coping style ($P = .05$, η^2 effect size: .11); no other differences between the groups were found ($P > .05$); • Effect sizes (η^2 .05–.06) tended to favor the MM group in seeking social support, on hostility and paranoid ideation scores (per authors, η^2 effect size: .01 = small, .06 = medium, .14 = large).	MQS: 8/17; CBS: −1 per ITT (−1 per PP) CES: −8 per ITT (−8 per PP) Groups were derived from separate residential facilities.
Case series						
Study 5. Zgierska et al. 2008 (53)	Relapse prevention in alcohol-dependent adults, graduates of the Intensive Outpatient Program	19 (10 F), mean age 38.4 (21–50 yrs); PSR 4.	Mindfulness-Based Relapse Prevention, 8 wks, therapist-led (120 min/wk) group sessions; based on the MBSR & MBCT programs, and Relapse Prevention Cognitive Therapy.	• Collected at 0, 4, 8, 12, 16 wks; • Alcohol use (self-report); • Severity of alcohol relapse triggers: stress, anxiety, depression, craving; • Salivary cortisol, serum IL-6, liver enzymes (0, 16 wks); • Meditation-related outcomes; Tx experiences.	• Retention: 78.9% PP: • During the study, HDD decreased ($p = .056$, ES .3), total number of drinks (ES .3) and PDA (ES .03) did not significantly change; • Stress, depression, anxiety severity improved ($P < .05$, ES .7–1.4); IL-6 level decreased ($P = .05$, ES .6); craving severity (ES .5), cortisol and liver enzymes levels did not significantly change; • Degree of mindfulness increased ($P < .05$, ES .7); all completers meditated at 16 wks, on average 4.6 days/wk during the study; • High Tx satisfaction; no adverse events.	MQS: 7/17; CBS: N/A per ITT (+1 per PP) The only study that directly reports (lack of) side effects and adverse events, and describes evaluating distributional characteristics of the data.

(Continued on next page)

TABLE 5. (Continued)

Study	Indication	Subjects	Intervention	Outcome measures	Results	Methodological quality/comments
Study 6. Davis et al. 2007 (50)	Smoking cessation, community setting	18 (10 F), mean age 45.2 (22–67 yrs); PSR 2; on average, subjects smoked 19.9 cigarettes/day for 26.4 yrs.	MBSR-based, with minor modifications, 8 wks, therapist-led group sessions (six 150 min/wk sessions + 1 7-hr retreat); quit date at wk 7 (after the retreat).	• Collected at 0–8 wks weekly, then 6 wks post-quit (12 wks post-entry); • Smoking (self-report, exhaled CO); • Stress, psychopathology symptom severity.	• Retention: 72% (however, 100% data collection rate for self-reported smoking). ITT = PP: • 10/18 (56%) quit smoking; PP: • Compared to nonquitters, those who quit meditated more ($P < .05$), with a possible dose-effect: 100% highly compliant, 40% moderately compliant, and 0% noncompliant meditators quit; • Compared to moderately compliant, highly compliant meditators decreased severity of stress one day post-quit ($P < .05$); baseline interest in meditation and affective distress were related to abstinence ($P < .05$).	MQS: 8/17; CBS: +2 per ITT (+2 per PP) Due to 100% data collection rate for the primary outcome, the primary analysis includes all subjects.
Study 7a. Bootzin & Stevens 2005 (49)	Sleep and sleepiness problems as relapse triggers among adolescents with SUDs	55 (21 F), age 13–19 yrs; PSR 3; adolescents with sleep or daytime sleepiness problems, graduates or graduating from outpatient addiction Tx programs.	MBSR-based, 7 wks, therapist-led five group sessions: 1st session—other interventions, not MBSR; 2nd–6th sessions—45 min MBSR + 45 min other Tx (stimulus control, bright light therapy, sleep hygiene, CT).	• Collected at 0–9 wks (weekly), 13, 52 wks; • Self-reported and objective sleep and sleepiness-related measures; • Self-reported substance use and psychological distress.	• Retention: 93%; PP: • drug use, low at baseline, increased during the Tx—no details provided; • Substance problem index plateaued for Tx completers (42% of the subjects), but it kept rising for those who did not complete Tx ($P < .2$, no details provided); • Sleep improved ($P < .05$) among Tx completers only; sleepiness, worry and mental health distress decreased during the study ($P < .05$).	MQS: 4/17; CBS: N/A per ITT (+2 per PP) Study focused on methods description; only preliminary results were reported, without details on substance use outcomes. Although the study intervention included MM, MM was not its primary focus.

Study	Research question	Sample	Intervention	Measures	Results	Methodological quality
Study 7b. Haynes et al. 2006 (57) (secondary analysis of Study 3a)	Is sleep improvement related to improved aggressive behavior among adolescents with SUDs	23 (13 F), mean age 16.4 (13–19 years); see Bootzin & Stevens 2005 (49) for other details.	See Bootzin & Stevens 2005 (49).	• See Bootzin & Stevens 2005 (49); • Two questions on presence or absence of aggressive thoughts or actions.	• Retention: 91%; PP: • Those reporting aggression at baseline, compared to others, had lower self-efficacy in resisting substance use urges ($P < .05$); • Post-Tx, those reporting aggression, compared to others, reported more frequent substance use, especially alcohol ($P < .05$); • All subjects improved some aspects of their sleep; poor sleep was related to aggression, after controlling for substance use.	See Bootzin & Stevens 2005 (49); Substance use was used as a covariate in the analysis, but was not the focus. No details on substance use are reported.
Study 7c. Stevens et al. 2007 (52) (secondary analysis of Study 3a)	Is sleep improvement related to improved trauma symptoms severity among adolescents with SUDs	20 (10 F), mean age 16.3 (13–19 years); see Bootzin & Stevens 2005 (49) for other details.	See Bootzin & Stevens 2005 (49)	• See Bootzin & Stevens 2005 (49); • Trauma Severity Index.	• Retention: unclear; PP: • Those with elevated trauma score at baseline, compared to others, had higher Substance Problem Index ($P < .05$). Substance use did not play a significant role in the analyses. • Those with better sleep characteristics had greater improvements in trauma scores than others.	See Bootzin & Stevens 2005 (49); Substance use was used as a covariate in the analysis, but was not the focus. No details on substance use are reported.
Study 8. Marcus et al. 2003 (51)	Stress severity among substance-dependent patients in residential Tx settings	21 (3 F), mean age 33.4 (21–51 yrs); PSR 4; therapeutic community patients with SUDs.	SOC + MBSR, 8 wks, therapist-led (150 min/wk) group sessions.	• Collected at 0, 8 wks; Salivary cortisol upon awakening; • Perceived Stress Scale.	• Retention: 85.7% (data collection rate: 57% cortisol, 76% surveys); PP: • Cortisol level decreased ($P < .05$, ES .65); • Perceived stress severity did not change ($P > .05$, ES .44).	MQS: 4/17; CBS: N/A per ITT (+1 PP) The study did not report substance use data.
Other studies						
Study 8: case report. Twohig et al. 2007 (54)	Marijuana dependence, community settings	3 (1 F), ages 19, 20, 43; PSR 2; marijuana dependent (5 were enrolled, 2 dropped out).	ACT, 8 wks, therapist-led (90 min/wk) individual therapy sessions.	• Collected at 0–8 wks (daily), and 13 wks; • Marijuana use (self-report, salivary swab); • Withdrawal severity, psychological outcomes.	• Retention: 3/5 (60%); • Although the 3 subjects did not use marijuana at 8 wks, they resumed its use by 13 wks (one to the pre-Tx level, and 2 at less than pre-Tx levels); • Withdrawal, anxiety and depression severity seemed to improve compared to baseline.	Methodological quality not scored. Manualized intervention.

(Continued on next page)

TABLE 5. (Continued)

Study	Indication	Subjects	Intervention	Outcome measures	Results	Methodological quality/comments
Study 9: qualitative study. Carroll et al. 2008 (56)	MBSR-related treatment experiences among substance-dependent patients in residential Tx settings	36 (6F), mean age 32.6 (19–54 yrs); PSR 4; residents of therapeutic community with SUDs.	MBSR, adapted to therapeutic community settings, 6 wks; therapist-led (180 min/wk) group sessions.	• 356 stories were reviewed (written as a part of guided expressive writing); • 38 stories of stress that referenced the MBSR therapy were identified and analyzed.	Analysis of 38 stories identified 3 main MBSR qualities: • Utility (usefulness for calming self, stress-reduction, coping); • Portability (ability to apply learned skills in real life), and • Sustainability (application of skills to a variety of different situations, goals).	This report was based on the ongoing unpublished trial. (72) Manualized intervention—the intervention description (MBSR for therapeutic community, MBSR-TC) was published elsewhere (87).
Study 10: qualitative study. Beitel et al. 2007 (55) (based on Margolin et al. 2006 (42) and 2007 (47) studies)	3-S treatment experience in methadone maintenance patients, a part of the studies by Margolin et al. 2006 (42) and 2007 (47)	39 (34 F), mean age 43 (28–54 yrs); PSR 4; opiate-dependent patients of methadone maintenance program, cocaine use disorder 77%, HIV-positive 38%.	3-S therapy: individual (46%) or individual + group (54%); see Margolin et al. 2006 (42) and 2007 (47) for details.	• Collected at post-Tx (8–12 wks post-entry); • Tx experiences questionnaire and interview.	• Preferred Tx format: 43% group, 14% individual, and 43% equally liked individual and group sessions; • all subjects meditated, on average 26 min/day; • 3-S was viewed as helpful for recovery, and different from the received SOC; • Meditation was the most liked and helpful aspect of the 3-S therapy; 49% reported a positive change resulting from 3-S therapy; subjects were satisfied with 3-S, and 97% would like to continue it; • No significant adverse events were reported.	See Margolin et al. 2006 (42) and 2007 (47) for details. Subjects did not describe any significant negative effects (side effects or adverse events) or problems associated with 3-S therapy.

Note. Results from the final follow-up are reported, unless stated otherwise.
Values (presented in [square brackets]) calculated for the systematic review: ARR: absolute risk reduction; CBS: Clinical Benefit Score; CES: Cumulative Evidence Score; ES: effect size (Cohen's *d*); MQS: Methodological Quality Score; NNT: number needed to treat; PSS: Population Severity Score.
CG: comparison group; CO: carbon monoxide; MM: mindfulness meditation; HIV: human immunodeficiency virus; ITT: intention to treat analysis; MBCT: Mindfulness-Based Cognitive Therapy; MBSR: Mindfulness-Based Stress Reduction; min: minutes; mos: months; NRT: nicotine replacement therapy; PP: per protocol analysis; PTSD: post-traumatic stress disorder; 3-S: Spiritual Self Schema; SOC: "standard of care" therapy; SUDs: substance use disorders; Tx: treatment; UTox: urine toxicology test; VM: Vipassana meditation; wks: weeks; yrs: years.

modified MBSR, with modifications being quite substantial and not manualized—therefore, these interventions were scored as "not manualized." Two studies developed and used an MBSR-based, manualized intervention: one patterned after MBSR and adjusted to the needs of therapeutic community residents (56) and one patterned after MBRP and adjusted to the needs of recovering, alcohol dependent adults (53). The meditation course intensity in the included studies ranged from five 90-minute sessions over 7 weeks (with less than 50% of the session content devoted to MM) (49,52,57) to eight 2-2.5-hour sessions over 8 weeks, with the majority of each session devoted to MM (36,43,46,50,53). In addition, 2 studies implemented a full-day retreat (36,50). Only one study reported monitoring the integrity of intervention delivery (56).

Spiritual Self Schema (3-S) therapy. The 3-S therapy has been developed for the treatment of addiction and human immunodeficiency virus (HIV) risk behavior (21). Its curriculum is manualized (www.3-S.us) and consists of an 8- or 12-week-long course, designed for clients at risk for, but not infected with, HIV or clients with HIV, respectively. The 3-S therapy teaches meditation and mindfulness skills in the context of comprehensive psychotherapy, integrating Buddhist principles with modern cognitive self-schema theory that is tailored to each patient's spiritual/religious faith (21).

Four reports (37,42,47,55), based on 3 separate studies (37,42,47), used manualized 3-S therapy delivered in an individual and/or group format, during 1- to 2-hour-long sessions per week, by a trained therapist over 8 (37,42,55) or 12 (47) weeks. Integrity of the intervention delivery was monitored in all the studies.

Acceptance and Commitment Therapy (ACT). Theoretically based in contemporary behavior analysis, ACT applies both mindfulness/acceptance, as well as commitment and behavior change processes (62). These core processes, conceptualized as positive psychological skills, aim to increase psychological flexibility that is defined as the ability to better connect to one's experience, and to make overt behavioral choices in the service of chosen goals and values ("committed action") (62). Originally developed for psychological disorders (20), ACT has

been applied to a variety of conditions, including SUDs.

Three studies used manualized ACT (38,39,54) delivered by a trained therapist in either an individual (54) or both individual and group (38,39) therapy format. The ACT sessions took place weekly, ranging in duration from $1^1/_2$ (54) to $3^1/_2$ (39) hours per week, over 7 (38) to 16 (39) weeks. Integrity of intervention delivery was monitored in all the studies.

Dialectical Behavior Therapy (DBT). DBT originated as a therapy for chronically suicidal clients with borderline personality disorder (19,70) and was subsequently adapted for SUDs (71). DBT comprises strategies from cognitive and behavioral therapies (with a problem-solving focus) and acceptance strategies (with mindfulness as its core) adapted from Zen teaching and practice. It provides a comprehensive long-term treatment that includes psychotherapy (therapist-led, in group, and individual formats) and case and medical management.

Two studies used a 1-year-long manualized DBT program for SUDs, with individual and group therapy lasting from 3 (41) to 6 (40) hours per week. Integrity of intervention delivery was monitored in these studies.

Methodological Quality

Randomization. All 7 RCTs (Table 4) received 4 points for randomization on the MQS scores, including the study that reported unequal effects of randomization (36)—in this case, a full MQS score was assigned since the "unequality" favored the controls. Two of the 7 RCTs used randomization techniques that require a comment. One of these RCTs initially randomized subjects into 2 arms: MM and "standard of care" control, and then subrandomized the MM group into 2 different protocols of MM delivery. Because no differences were found between the 2 MM subgroups, they were later combined into 1 group for the final analysis, and compared to controls (42). Another RCT randomly assigned subjects to 2 different modes of MM delivery, but found no differences between these groups (no details described); thus, the groups were combined into one, and assessed as a prospective case series, with detailed results presented for pre-post analyses only (37).

Blinding. "Double-blinding" and interventionist or subject blinding are not feasible and/or desirable in studies using MM interventions for practical and ethical reasons, and none of the treatment studies used such methods. Three RCTs reported assessor blinding (39–41).

Sample size. The included studies were "pilots" with small sample sizes. One published RCT (39) and one unpublished RCT (59) provided sample size assumptions; however, a high attrition rate resulted in their being underpowered.

Analysis. Only one study described evaluation of the distributional characteristics of the variables, and the use of parametric or nonparametric tests, when appropriate (53). One published study (43) and one unpublished study (58) did not use statistical analyses for the assessment of intervention effects. Other studies used parametric analyses that assume normal data distribution. However, in the context of small sample sizes and high variability of some data (as indicated by SDs), it is possible that some variables did not have normal distribution. Six studies reported 100% follow-up data collection (50), 100% retention (46), or analyzed data per intention-to-treat (ITT) protocol, imputing missing data (38–41).

Quality of MM intervention delivery. MM was manualized in 15 separate studies, described in 18 articles (37–48,50,51,53–56). Integrity of the intervention delivery (therapist protocol adherence and/or competence) was monitored in 10 separate studies (37–42,47,50,54,56).

Retention rate. Retention rate among the MM subjects ranged from about 45% (39,44) to 100% (46), with an average rate of 75%. One study with a 72% retention rate collected primary outcome data for all enrolled subjects (50).

Methodological Quality Score (MQS) and Cumulative Evidence Score (CES) (Table 3). Among the included 22 reports, 15 controlled trials or prospective case series were based on separate studies. As expected, among these 15 studies, the highest MQSs were for RCTs, followed by nonrandomized controlled trials and case series. Only one RCT (40) received a score of "excellent," defined as MQS ≥ 14 (23). Eval-

uating by the type of MM intervention used, the highest MQSs were achieved by studies of DBT and ACT, followed by 3-S and MBSR-based therapies. The MBSR-based intervention was the most commonly studied MM therapy (7/15 studies). Grouping by subject population, the highest mean MQSs were achieved by studies evaluating adults with SUDs in the outpatient setting, which were also the most common population/settings (N = 7: opiate dependent, medically managed subjects—5 studies; poly-SUDs—1 study; and alcohol dependence—1 study); these studies were followed by studies of community-recruited adults with tobacco dependence (N = 3), and studies of adults treated for SUDs in residential settings (N = 3). The Overall CES, calculated for subgroups of studies, indicated that, in general, the studies yielded positive evidence (Overall CES ranging from +10 to +143), with 50% to 85% of the studies reporting positive outcomes by ITT (N = 6) or per protocol (N = 13) analyses, respectively (Table 3).

Side Effects or Adverse Events

Only 2 reports directly stated that no MM-related significant side effects, adverse events, or problems occurred (53,55). Other reports did not address this topic, implicitly suggesting lack of negative effects.

Results of the Published Treatment RCTs (Table 4)

Seven RCTs, including a total of 383 (63% female) adult subjects, followed for an average of 38 weeks post-entry (from 8 (37,42) to 68 (40,41) weeks), offered the most detailed assessment of MM interventions. Methodological quality of the RCTs was moderate (MQS 8-14/17). Six RCTs evaluated severely impaired populations (PSR 4/4), and one (38) focused on tobacco dependent adults (PSR 2/4).

Six of 7 RCTs used a 2-arm, and 1 used a 3-arm design (39). Three studies compared MM + "standard of care" (SOC) to SOC alone (36,42), with both MM and SOC provided at the same clinical site. One study compared MM to SOC, with SOC subjects referred out for therapy ("naturalistic control") (41). Finally, 4 studies

(37–40) compared MM to an active intervention: 3 to a different therapy (behavioral (39,40) or pharmacotherapy (38)) and 1 compared MM delivered in "individual" versus "individual + group format" (37).

All RCTs reported some positive results. Compared to SOC, the MM intervention showed positive effects as indicated by the ITT (40,41) and per protocol (38–42) analyses. Differential improvement in both substance use-related and other outcomes was noted in 5 of 7 studies (38–42). One study (36) noted a differential improvement in medical symptom severity only ($P < .05$, effect size .2), and one study (37) comparing 3-S "individual" to 3-S "individual + group" therapy did not find differences between the study arms, but noted pre-post improvements ($P < .05$, effect size .5) in substance use outcomes.

Overall, studies using SOC (39,41,42) or active, but "nonmatching" interventions (38) as a comparison group, tended to report greater statistically significant between-group differences, with results favoring MM, than studies using a "matching" behavioral intervention (39,40) The 3-arm study by Hayes and colleagues (39), with the largest sample size but low retention rate, of 124 poly-substance–abusing methadone maintenance patients suggested, in a per protocol analysis, that MM + SOC may result in a substantial reduction of substance use compared to SOC alone (ARR 33%). This finding was consistent across 3 other RCTs comparing MM to SOC (ARR 30% (42) with medium to large effect size (41)) or to pharmacotherapy with medical management (ARR 12% to 20% per ITT and per protocol analyses) (38). Two methodologically strong RCTs compared MM to a different behavioral intervention that "matched" MM by subject involvement and therapy format (39,40). These studies did not find significant in-between group differences in substance use (ARR 5% to 12%; $P > .05$) or psychological outcomes at the study end point at 42 (39) or 68 (40) weeks; however, they both noted a tendency to a more accurate drug use reporting among MM compared to comparison subjects (39,40). Regarding non–substance use–related measures, MM subjects, compared to SOC controls, increased their motivation for HIV prevention, their spiritual practices, and showed a cognitive shift from "addict"

to "spiritual qualities" ($P < .05$) (42); they also improved their Global Adjustment and Global Social Adjustment Scale scores ($P < .05$) (41).

Results of the Published Nonrandomized Controlled Studies, Case Reports, and Case Series (Table 5)

Table 5 summarizes 4 controlled nonrandomized trials (described by 6 articles (43–48)), 4 case series (described by 6 articles (49–53,57)), and 1 case report (54). These studies included 609 subjects, 13 to 67 years old, suffering from various SUDs, and recruited from the outpatient treatment (46,47,49,51–53,57), community (43,50), or jail (44,48) settings.

Although the methodological quality of the scored studies was limited (MQS 4–8/17), collectively they reported overall positive outcomes. On average, substance use tended to decrease at follow-up compared to baseline (43,50,53) or compared to a control group (44,47), with effect sizes ranging from small (47,53) to medium (44). One study (49) reported an increase in substance use at follow-up compared to low-use at baseline, but no detailed results were presented, and substance use was not the primary focus of the study. Severity of potential relapse triggers (such as stress, mental health and sleep problems, certain coping styles) also tended to improve compared to both baseline (49,50,53) and control conditions (44,46,47), and the average effect size for these changes ranged from medium to large. Bowen and colleagues (44) also noted a reduction of alcohol-related negative consequences (small effect size) among subjects who underwent MM training compared to controls. Only one uncontrolled trial (among all included studies) of alcoholics treated with MM therapy, adjunctive to SOC, assessed craving severity and the degree of mindfulness (53). Although craving severity decreased (medium effect size), this change was not statistically significant; degree of mindfulness, or the ability to be attentive to a present-moment experience in daily life, improved (medium effect size), and this change correlated to decreased stress severity (large effect size) at 16-week follow-up (53).

Participation in the MM therapy correlated to or mediated the improvements in substance use and relapse-related outcomes, with small-to-large effect size (44,45,47,48,50,53). One uncontrolled study compared "relapsers" ($N = 7$; subjects reporting at least one heavy drinking day during the study) to "nonrelapsers" ($N = 8$), and found that relapsers had more severe symptoms of anxiety, depression, and craving, reported lower degree of mindfulness, and meditated fewer minutes per day ($P < .05$) (53). The same study also reported that drinking level as well as the change in drinking correlated to the severity of relapse risk factors such as anxiety, depression, stress, and craving (large effect sizes) and the change in their severity, respectively. In turn, severity of relapse risk factors negatively correlated with the intensity of a daily meditation practice (large effect size) (53).

Two uncontrolled trials assessed pre-post levels of biological outcomes: stress-responsive and illness-sensitive biomarkers, in addition to self-reported psychological measures. A study of recovering alcoholics evaluated serum interleukin-6 (IL-6), liver enzymes, and diurnal profile of salivary cortisol at baseline and 16-week follow-up (53). Whereas cortisol ($N = 10$) and liver enzymes ($N = 12$) did not significantly change over time (small effect size), IL-6 level decreased ($N = 12$; medium effect size, $P = .05$), suggesting a reduction in chronic stress level and improved health. After MM intervention, SUD-affected residents of a therapeutic community showed a decrease in an awakening salivary cortisol level compared to baseline (medium effect size) (51).

Subject Treatment Experiences Related to MM Intervention (Tables 4 and 5)

Two qualitative studies (55,56), derived from mixed-methods primary projects (42,47,72), focused on subject treatment experiences related to MM therapy (Table 5). Several other studies also evaluated subject experiences, using quantitative (e.g., Likert scales) or qualitative techniques (38,39,43,53). Taken together, MM therapy was well received by the subjects with different degrees of problem severity (PSR 2–4/4) and in various settings: residential (56), outpatient (39,53,55), and community (38,43). Subjects reported high degree of satisfaction

with MM therapy and its usefulness as a recovery-enhancing tool. They also viewed MM-related skills as unique, "brand new," and different from those taught in a traditional, professional addiction treatment (53,55).

Four studies evaluated individual ("at-home") MM practices among the subjects who underwent an 8-week MM intervention (36,42,43,53). Two of these studies, using the MBSR-based intervention, reported that about 47% of the subjects continued meditation practice at 12 (43) and 22 (36) weeks post-entry. A study evaluating MBSR + CBT–based intervention found that 100% of the study completers (79% of the sample, with all drop-outs occurring after the first or second MM session) meditated at 16 weeks, on average 3.9 days/week, 27.4 minutes/meditating day (53). Likewise, an RCT evaluating 3-S therapy found that at 8 weeks, all study completers (82%) continued meditating, on average 26 minutes/day (42).

Unpublished Studies (Table 6)

Two treatment trials using ACT (58,59) and one laboratory-based study of a mindfulness-based coping technique (60) provide additional insights into the potential efficacy and mechanisms of MM interventions for smoking cessation. An RCT of 10-week MM intervention (ACT, combined with CBT and nicotine replacement therapy [NRT]) found a significantly higher quit rate (small effect size) and higher treatment satisfaction (medium effect size) among the MM subjects compared to controls, receiving NRT alone, at 52 weeks; in addition, acceptance-based responding mediated effects of MM on smoking outcomes (59). A set of prospective case series ($N = 16$ subjects), designed for pilot-testing and refinement of the study methods, evaluated effects of combined ACT, CBT, and NRT. Although smoking quantity and frequency have not been compared "prepost," and all study completers resumed smoking at 26 weeks post quit date, the longest continuous abstinence period was longer after the MM intervention than during subjects' previous attempts when abstinence had lasted less than 3 days. Further, 82% of the subjects reported that they learned skills that were "very" or

TABLE 6. Unpublished Treatment Trials and a Laboratory-Based Study of Mindfulness or Mindfulness Meditation Based Interventions (MM) Used for the Treatment of Substance Use, Misuse, or Disorders: Methods and Results

Study	Design and indication	Subjects	Intervention	Outcome measures	Results	MQS
Study 1. Gifford et al. 2008, submitted (59)	2-Arm RCT: smoking cessation, community settings	303 (10 F), mean age 46.0 (18–75 yrs); PSR 2; tobacco-dependent, community-recruited adults; on average, 24 cigarettes/day.	• MM intervention, 10 wks: ACT + Functional Analytic Psychotherapy (therapist-led, weekly 120-min group and 50-min individual sessions) + bupropion. • CG: bupropion only (medical management, one 60-min educational meeting, handouts)	• Collected at 0, 10, 26, 52 wks; • Smoking (7-day point prevalence; self-report, exhaled CO); • Withdrawal severity, psychological health; • Tx experience.	• Retention: 45.2%; PP: • Quit rate was higher at the MM than control group (31.6% vs. 17.5%, $P < .05$, ES .3 [ARR 14.1, NNT 7]); • During 52 wks, MM was more effective in reducing smoking than control Tx (OR 2.2, $P < .05$); • Acceptance-based responding and the therapeutic relationship mediated effects of MM on Tx outcomes; • MM group reported higher Tx satisfaction than controls at all time points ($P < .05$, ES .7 at 52 wks).	MQS: 10/17; CBS: N/A per ITT (+2 per PP) Manualized MM intervention.
Study 2. Brown et al. 2008* submitted (58)	Case series: smoking cessation, community settings	16 (12 F), mean age 41.9 (18–65 yrs); PSR 2; tobacco-dependent, community-recruited adults; on average, 20.4 cigarettes/day.	• MM intervention, 10 wks, therapist-led: ACT + cognitive behavioral therapy (wks 4–10) + NRT (wks 6–14).	• Collected at 0, 10, 14, 19, 32 wks (quit date: week 6); • Smoking (self-reported, exhaled CO); • Withdrawal and depressive symptom severity.	• Retention: 75%; • Quit rates at 10, 14, 19, 32 wks: 31%, 25%, 19%, and 0%. • During the study, the longest continuous abstinence was median 24 days (mean 41.6), number of days abstinent was median 40.5 (mean 58.8, out of 180 study days), time to relapse (7 consecutive smoking days) was median 45.5 days (mean 49.9), and number of quit-smoking attempts was median 2.5 times (mean 4.1). • 82% reported that the learned skills were "very" or "extremely useful" in helping quit smoking.	MQS: 5/17; CBS: N/A Since no statistical assessment of the significance of pre-post change was provided; only descriptive statistics were used. Follow-up psychological outcomes were not reported. Manualized intervention.

(Continued on next page)

TABLE 6. (Continued)

Study	Design and indication	Subjects	Intervention	Outcome measures	Results	MQS
Study 3. Bowen 2008, PhD dissertation (60)	2-Arm RCT, laboratory study; smoking, related craving and negative affect; community settings	123 (34 F), mean age 20.3 (18–46 yrs); PSR 2; undergraduate psychology students; on average, low dependence scores, smoked 5.3 cigarettes/day in the past week.	Subjects did not smoke for 12 hrs prior, then underwent 4 brief cue (cigarette) exposures in a 90-min long laboratory session, during which they were asked to cope using: • MM intervention (n = 61): guided, audio-recorded, mindfulness-based strategies; • CG (n = 62): their "usual" coping strategies.	• Collected post-exposure (4 in-person assessments), at 1 and 7 days; • Smoking (self-reported); • Smoking urges, affect; • Brief written description of used coping strategies.	• Retention: 90.2%; PP: • During the follow-up week, MM group smoked fewer cigarettes/day than controls ($P < .05$, ES .6); compared to baseline, MM decreased smoking by 26%, whereas CG increased it by 11%; • No significant differences between groups were found in latency to the first cigarette, negative affect and smoking urges; • During cue exposures, to cope with cravings and urges, MM group used MM strategies, whereas controls used primarily distraction-based techniques.	MQS: 9/17; CBS: N/A per ITT (+2 per PP) Manualized intervention.

Note. Results from the final follow-up are reported, unless stated otherwise.

*Since completion of this review, a report from this study has been published (61).

Values (presented in [square brackets]) calculated for the systematic review: ARR: absolute risk reduction; CBS: Clinical Benefit Score; CES: Cumulative Evidence Score; ES: effect size (Cohen's *d*); MQS: Methodological Quality Score; NNT: number needed to treat; PSS: Population Severity Score.

ACT: Acceptance Commitment Therapy; CO: carbon monoxide; MM: mindfulness meditation; ITT: intention to treat analysis; min: minutes; mos: months; NRT: nicotine replacement therapy; PP: per protocol analysis; Tx: treatment; UTox: urine toxicology test; wks: weeks; yrs: years.

"extremely useful" in helping them quit smoking (58). Finally, one RCT (PhD dissertation) described an experiment evaluating efficacy of mindfulness-based coping compared to "usual" coping strategies aimed to prevent relapse after quitting smoking (60). In this study, during a cue exposure paradigm, the MM group used MM strategies, as instructed, whereas controls used primarily distraction-based techniques to cope with smoking cravings and urges. During the 7-day follow-up, the MM group smoked fewer cigarettes/day than controls (medium effect size, $P < .05$). Overall, the results of these unpublished trials support the existing preliminary evidence provided by published studies.

DISCUSSION

This is the first systematic review of mindfulness or mindfulness meditation–based interventions (MM) for substance use, misuse, or disorders. Although existing data are preliminary and do not allow a consensus recommendation for any particular type of MM intervention for any single substance use–related condition, several findings are of clinical, theoretical, and research interest.

The majority of the reviewed studies showed some positive outcomes among SUD-affected subjects treated with MM intervention, compared to baseline or other therapy (most commonly SOC). The case studies illustrated how MM had been practiced from a historical and clinical perspective. The focus on real-life trial methods has been termed pragmatic (73). Pragmatic studies have the advantage of assessing effectiveness under conditions that patients encounter in real-life settings, thereby avoiding confounders associated with highly standardized clinical trial settings. Though lacking methodological strengths of control and randomization, the case studies, documented here, consistently showed positive patient outcomes and the general treatment satisfaction of subjects with chronic, often refractory, SUDs who were treated with MM therapy. Pragmatic aspects of these studies included meeting patient's expectations of receiving a "promised treatment," the ability of the therapist to better select the patient,

and study methods that more closely resemble real clinical settings. Data from the controlled trials suggest that subjects receiving MM, adjunctive to SOC or pharmacotherapy, do as well or better than those receiving SOC or pharmacotherapy alone. When compared to other behavioral interventions in RCT settings, MM appears to produce comparable results. All these conclusions require assessment with more formal methodology in adequately powered clinical trials.

The promise of MM as an efficacious treatment for SUDs is supported by the consistency of positive results, demonstrated in this review across different study designs, MM modalities, subject populations, and addictive disorders treated. Additional support for the potential efficacy of MM in SUDs can be drawn from the results of studies of other clinical samples. MM-based therapies have been shown to be effective or potentially effective (with, on average, medium pooled effect size, Cohen's d .5 to .7 (16,62)) for a variety of medical and mental health disorders, including stress, anxiety, depression, emotion dysregulation, and avoidance coping (16,62,74–77), all known risk factors for relapse in SUDs (78,79). In this context, MM may be particularly helpful for patients with co-occurring substance use and mental health disorders ("dual diagnosis").

Although long-term MM practice patterns have not been assessed in the context of SUDs, its use in other clinical samples suggests that MM can have long-lasting effects. For example, after a meditation course, 60% to 90% of subjects still meditated up to 4 years later, and reported that the course "had lasting value" and was highly important (16). Patient satisfaction is an important consideration when choosing between treatment alternatives (80). MM also appears safe—rigorous studies have not reported any side effects or adverse events (64,65). This review corroborates these findings.

It is appealing to assume that the preliminary positive results in MM studies are direct outcomes of MM interventions; however, such a hypothesis is premature. The theoretical framework behind MM as well as early indirect evidence supports the use of MM for SUDs (8,9,13,14) and suggests unique therapeutic properties of MM. On a conceptual level, MM stands out as distinctive and, in many ways, different from other existing behavioral modalities, specifically from cognitive behavioral therapy (CBT), which is commonly used to treat SUDs (81,82). Whereas CBT promotes adaptive, antecedent-focused coping strategies (e.g., targeting emotion cues), meditation targets maladaptive, response-focused strategies, such as emotional avoidance, suppression, or impulse control; thus, MM-related skills can complement skills acquired through CBT (8,9,13,14). The integration of meditation and traditional CBT strategies may improve overall treatment efficacy, e.g., by increasing awareness of sensations, such as craving, emotional states, and physiological arousal (83). Recent pilot trials of clinical cohorts add support to the above hypotheses, indicating that MM and CBT can produce different effects on mental health outcomes (62,84,85). Two reviewed qualitative studies (53,55) reported that subjects viewed MM-related skills as different from those acquired through "traditional" SOC therapy for addiction.

Limitations of this review include limiting the inclusion criteria to studies published in English, potentially excluding relevant studies. Lack of reviewer blinding and lack of assessment of inter-rater agreement could have introduced bias. Although the included interventions were based on the MM principles, they were heterogeneous; evaluating them together as one "MM intervention" could have introduced bias.

Strengths of this review include an exhaustive literature search and application of statistical methods allowing direct comparison of included studies.

Directions for further research. Existing studies of MM therapy for addictive disorders are far from definitive and the research methods are evolving. These clinical and research fields would benefit from the development of (1) standardized scientific parameters to be used in future studies of MM as a therapy for addictive disorders; (2) a comprehensive conceptual model of possible mechanisms underlying MM efficacy in SUDs; and (3) recommendations on MM implementation in clinical addiction medicine settings. Below we elaborate on each of these recommendations:

1. Research methods of MM studies in addiction settings require refinement and standardization.
   - A written manual should be used to guide the meditation intervention. It has been suggested that best therapeutic effects are achieved when the meditation intervention is adjusted to accommodate the specific needs of the targeted population (86). Several "manualized" MM therapies are currently used in the treatment of SUDs (MBSR, MBRP, DBT, ACT, 3-S), most have been modified and adjusted to the needs of individual studies; however, only a minority of these studies developed a separate intervention manual. It is not known whether even relatively minor adaptations could have affected outcomes. Standardization of treatment manuals would facilitate study replication and data pooling.
   - A theory for, and measures to assess, the evaluation of treatment outcomes in the context of MM also require development.
   - Assessment of subjects' MM practice intensity and changes in the degree of mindfulness should be considered. These are essentially the "dose" and "quality" of the intervention and as such have the potential to influence findings similar to medication dose-response effects in pharmacotherapy trials. These data would also provide information on the ability of subjects to sustain MM practice over time. Many clinical MM programs "interview" potential clients before enrollment to ensure appropriate selection. In research settings, including the reviewed studies, the eligibility criteria are usually diagnosis-driven; results may therefore be skewed away from a positive effect, should one exist.
2. Research of MM has the potential to create a comprehensive bench-to-bedside explanatory model of its effects. Therefore, the mechanism of MM should be assessed in tandem with clinical assessment. Possible mechanisms have been hypothesized (8,9,13,14); however, no comprehensive model, encompassing biopsychological aspects of addiction, has been developed. None of the included studies was designed as

a "dismantling" study or focused on "active ingredients" underlying MM effects. Appropriate control therapies and targeted assessments, including "objective" measures (e.g., biomarkers, imaging studies) are needed to assess treatment efficacy and to elucidate a mechanism of action for MM interventions in addictive disorders.

3. Although MM techniques are already used in the clinical setting to treat addictive disorders (14), it is premature to formally recommend for or against such practice. Researchers and clinicians involved in MM research should collectively address effectiveness of MM therapies in the form of consensus statements, and thereby provide guidelines on the best ways to implement MM therapies in clinical settings as a part of comprehensive addiction treatment programs.

CONCLUSIONS

Conclusive data for MM as a treatment for addictive disorders are lacking. However, the preliminary evidence suggests MM efficacy. MM therapies appear safe when performed in clinical research settings. Significant methodological limitations exist in most studies published to date, and it is unclear which persons with addictive disorders might benefit most from MM. Future clinical trials must be of sufficient sample size to answer a specific clinical question and should include carefully designed comparison groups that would allow assessment of both the effect size and mechanism of action of MM.

REFERENCES

1. United Nations Office of Drugs and Crime (UNODC). *Global Illicit Drug Trends 2007*. New York: United Nations; 2007.

2. Substance Abuse and Mental Health Services Administration (SAMHSA), Office of Applied Studies. Results from the 2005 National Survey on Drug Use and Health: Detailed Tables; Prevalence Estimates, Standard Errors, P Values, and Sample Sizes. September 2006. http:/www.oas.samhsa.gov (accessed Jun 9, 2007).

3. Office of National Drug Control Policy (ONDCP). *The Economic Costs of Drug Abuse in the United States 1992–2002*. Washington, DC: ONDCP; 2004.

4. Connors GJ, Maisto SA, Donovan DM. Conceptualizations of relapse: a summary of psychological and psychobiological models. *Addiction.* 1996;91(Suppl):S5–S13.

5. Mackay PW, Marlatt GA. Maintaining sobriety: stopping is starting. *Int J Addict.* 1990;25:1257–1276.

6. Miller WR, Walters ST, Bennett ME. How effective is alcoholism treatment in the United States? *J Stud Alcohol.* 2001;62:211–220.

7. Marlatt GA, Grodon JR. *Relapse prevention: Maintenance Strategies in the Treatment of Addictive Behaviors.* New York: Guilford Press; 1985.

8. Breslin FC, Zach M, McMain S. An information-processing analysis of mindfulness: implications for relapse prevention in the treatment of substance abuse. *Clin Psychol Sci Prac.* 2002;9:275–299.

9. Marlatt GA, Chawla N. Meditation and alcohol use. *South Med J.* 2007;100:451–453.

10. Kabat-Zinn J. *Full Catastrophe Living: Using the Wisdom of Your Body and Mind to Face Stress, Pain, and Illness.* New York: Delta; 1990.

11. Kabat-Zinn J. An outpatient program in behavioral medicine for chronic pain patients based on the practice of mindfulness meditation: theoretical considerations and preliminary results. *Gen Hosp Psychiatry.* 1982;4:33–47.

12. Kutz I, Borysenko JZ, Benson H. Meditation and psychotherapy: a rationale for the integration of dynamic psychotherapy, the relaxation response, and mindfulness meditation. *Am J Psychiatry.* 1985;142:1–8.

13. Hofmann SG, Asmundson GJ. Acceptance and mindfulness-based therapy: new wave or old hat? *Clin Psychol Rev.* 2008;28:1–16.

14. Hoppes K. The application of mindfulness-based cognitive interventions in the treatment of co-occurring addictive and mood disorders. *CNS Spectr.* 2006;11:829–851.

15. Salmon PG, Santorelli SF, Kabat-Zinn J. Intervention elements promoting adherence to mindfulness-based stress reduction programs in the clinical behavioral medicine setting. In: Schumacher SM, et al., eds. *Handbook of Health Behavior Change.* New York: Springer; 1998:239–268.

16. Baer RA. Mindfulness training as a clinical intervention: a conceptual and empirical review. *Clin Psychol Sci Prac.* 2003;10:125–143.

17. Segal ZV, Williams JM, Teasdale JD. *Mindfulness-based Cognitive Therapy for Depression: A New Approach to Preventing Relapse.* New York: Guilford Publications; 2002.

18. Witkiewitz K, Marlatt GA. Mindfulness-based relapse prevention for alcohol and substance use disorders: the meditative tortoise wins the race. *J Cognit Psychother.* 2005;19:221–230.

19. Linehan MM. *Cognitive-Behavioral Treatment of Borderline Personality Disorder.* New York: Guilford; 1993.

20. Hayes SC, Strosahl KD, Wilson KG. *Acceptance and Commitment Therapy: An Experimental Approach to Behavior Change.* New York, Guilford Press; 1999.

21. Avants SK, Margolin A. Development of Spiritual Self-Schema Therapy for the treatment of addictive and HIV risk behavior: a convergence of cognitive and Buddhist psychology. *J Psychother Integr.* 2004;14:253–289.

22. Manheimer E, Anderson BJ, Stein MD. Use and assessment of complementary and alternative therapies by intravenous drug users. *Am J Drug Alcohol Abuse.* 2003;29:401–413.

23. Miller RM, Wilbourne PL, Hettema JE. What works? A summary of alcohol treatment outcome research. In: Hester RK, Miller WR, eds. *Handbook of Alcoholism Treatment Approaches.* 3rd ed. Boston: Allyn & Bacon; 2003. Scoring manual available at http://casaa.unm.edu/download/mesa.pdf2003.

24. Cropley M, Ussher M, Charitou E. Acute effects of a guided relaxation routine (body scan) on tobacco withdrawal symptoms and cravings in abstinent smokers. *Addiction.* 2007;102:989–993.

25. Drummond DC, Glautier S. A controlled trial of cue exposure treatment in alcohol dependence. *J Consult Clin Psychol.* 1994;62:809–817.

26. Gilbert GS, Parker JC, Claiborn CD. Differential mood changes in alcoholics as a function of anxiety management strategies. *J Clin Psychol.* 1978;34:229–232.

27. McIver S, O'Halloran P, McGartland M. The impact of Hatha yoga on smoking behavior. *Altern Ther Health Med.* 2004;10:22–23.

28. Niederman R. The effects of Chi-Kung on spirituality and alcohol/other drug dependency recovery. *Alcohol Treat Q.* 2003;21:22–23.

29. Parker JC, Gilbert GS, Thoreson RW. Reduction of autonomic arousal in alcoholics: a comparison of relaxation and meditation techniques. *J Consult Clin Psychol.* 1978;46:879–886.

30. Rohsenow DJ, Monti PM, Martin RA, Colby SM, Myers MG, Gulliver SB, Brown RA, Mueller TI, Gordon A, Abrams DB. Motivational enhancement and coping skills training for cocaine abusers: effects on substance use outcomes. *Addiction.* 2004;99:862–874.

31. Rohsenow DJ, Monti PM, Rubonis AV, Gulliver SB, Colby SM, Binkoff JA, Abrams DB. Cue exposure with coping skills training and communication skills training for alcohol dependence: 6- and 12-month outcomes. *Addiction.* 2001;96:1161–1174.

32. Rohsenow DJ, Smith RE, Johnson S. Stress management training as a prevention program for heavy social drinkers: cognitions, affect, drinking, and individual differences. *Addict Behav.* 1985;10:45–54.

33. Shaffer HJ, LaSalvia TA, Stein JP. Comparing Hatha yoga with dynamic group psychotherapy for enhancing methadone maintenance treatment: a randomized clinical trial. *Altern Ther Health Med.* 1997;3:57–66.

34. Ussher M, West R, Doshi R, Sampuran AK. Acute effect of isometric exercise on desire to smoke and tobacco withdrawal symptoms. *Hum Psychopharmacol.* 2006;21:39–46.

35. Rohsenow DJ, Monti PM, Martin RA, Michalec E, Abrams DB. Brief coping skills treatment for cocaine abuse: 12-month substance use outcomes. *J Consult Clin Psychol.* 2000;68:515–520.

36. Alterman AI, Koppenhaver JM, Mulholland E, Ladden LJ, Baime MJ. Pilot trial of effectiveness of mindfulness meditation for substance abuse patients. *J Subst Use.* 2004;9:259–268.

37. Avants SK, Beitel M, Margolin A. Making the shift from 'addict self' to 'spiritual self.' Results from a Stage 1 study of Spritual Self-Schema (3-S) therapy for the treatment of addiction and HIV risk behavior. *Mental Health Religion Culture.* 2005;8:167–177.

38. Gifford EV, Kohlenberg BS, Hayes SC, Antonuccio DO, Piasecki M, Rasmussen-Hall ML, Palm KM. Acceptance-based treatment for smoking cessation. *Behav Ther.* 2004;35:689–705.

39. Hayes SC, Wilson KG, Gifford EV, Bissett R, Piasecki M, Batten S, Byrd M, Gregg J. A preliminary trial of twelve-step facilitation and acceptance and commtiment therapy with polysubstance-abusing methadone-maintained opiate addicts. *Behav Ther.* 2004;35:667–688.

40. Linehan MM, Dimeff LA, Reynolds SK, Comtois KA, Welch SS, Heagerty P, Kivlahan DR. Dialectical behavior therapy versus comprehensive validation therapy plus 12-step for the treatment of opioid dependent women meeting criteria for borderline personality disorder. *Drug Alcohol Depend.* 2002;67:13–26.

41. Linehan MM, Schmidt H, 3rd, Dimeff LA, Craft JC, Kanter J, Comtois KA. Dialectical behavior therapy for patients with borderline personality disorder and drug-dependence. *Am J Addict.* 1999;8:279–292.

42. Margolin A, Beitel M, Schuman-Olivier Z, Avants SK. A controlled study of a spiritually-focused intervention for increasing motivation for HIV prevention among drug users. *AIDS Educ Prevent.* 2006;18:311–322.

43. Altner N. Mindfulness practice and smoking cessation: The Essen Hospital Smoking Cessation Study (EASY). *J Meditat Meditat Res.* 2002;1:9–18.

44. Bowen S, Witkiewitz K, Dillworth TM, Chawla N, Simpson TL, Ostafin BD, Larimer ME, Blume AW, Parks GA, Marlatt GA. Mindfulness meditation and substance use in an incarcerated population. *Psychol Addict Behav.* 2006;20:343–347.

45. Bowen S, Witkiewitz K, Dillworth TM, Marlatt GA. The role of thought suppression in the relationship between mindfulness meditation and alcohol use. *Addict Behav.* 2007;32:2324–2328.

46. Marcus MT, Fine M, Kouzekanani K. Mindfulness-based meditation in a therapeutic community. *J Subst Use.* 2001;5:305–311.

47. Margolin A, Schuman-Olivier Z, Beitel M, Arnold A, Fulwiler CE, Avants SK. A preliminary study of Spiritual Self-Schema (3-S) therapy for reducing impulsivity in HIV-positive drug users. *J Clin Psychol.* 2007;63:979–999.

48. Simpson TL, Kaysen D, Bowen S, MacPherson LM, Chawla N, Blume A, Marlatt GA, Larimer M. PTSD symptoms, substance use, and vipassana meditation among incarcerated individuals. *J Trauma Stress*. 2007;20:239–249.

49. Bootzin RR, Stevens SJ. Adolescents, substance abuse, and the treatment of insomnia and daytime sleepiness. *Clin Psychol Rev*. 2005;25:629–644.

50. Davis JM, Fleming MF, Bonus KA, Baker TB. A pilot study on mindfulness based stress reduction for smokers. *BMC Complement Altern Med*. 2007;7:2.

51. Marcus MT, Fine M, Moeller FG, Khan MM, Pitts K, Swank PR, Liehr P. Change in stress levels following mindfulness-based stress reduction in a therapeutic community. *Addict Disord Treat*. 2003;2:63–68.

52. Stevens S, Haynes PL, Ruiz B, Bootzin RR. Effects of a behavioral sleep medicine intervention on trauma symptoms in adolescents recently treated for substance abuse. *Subst Abuse*. 2007;28:21–31.

53. Zgierska A, Rabago D, Zuelsdorff M, Coe C, Miller M, Fleming M. Mindfulness meditation for alcohol relapse prevention: a feasibility pilot study. *J Addict Med*. 2008;2:165–173.

54. Twohig MP, Shoenberger D, Hayes SC. A preliminary investigation of acceptance and commitment therapy as a treatment for marijuana dependence in adults. *J Appl Behav Anal*. 2007;40:619–632.

55. Beitel M, Genova M, Schuman-Olivier Z, Arnold R, Avants SK, Margolin A. Reflections by inner-city drug users on a Buddhist-based spirituality-focused therapy: a qualitative study. *Am J Orthopsychiatry*. 2007;77:1–9.

56. Carroll D, Lange B, Liehr P, Raines S, Marcus MT. Evaluating Mindfulness-Based Stress Reduction: analyzing stories of stress to formulate focus group questions. *Arch Psychiatr Nurs*. 2008;22:107–109.

57. Haynes PL, Bootzin RR, Smith L, Cousins J, Cameron M, Stevens S. Sleep and aggression in substance-abusing adolescents: results from an integrative behavioral sleep-treatment pilot program. *Sleep*. 2006;29:512–520.

58. Brown RA, Palm KM, Strong DR, Lejuez CW, Kahler CW, Zvolensky MJ, Hayes SC, Wilson KG, Gifford EV. Distress tolerance treatment for early-lapse smokers: rationale, program description, and preliminary findings. *In preparation*, 2008. (See reference 61.)

59. Gifford EV, et al. Applying acceptance and the therapeutic relationship to smoking cessation: a randomized controlled trial. *In preparation*. 2008.

60. Bowen S. Effects of Mindfulness-Based Instructions on Negative Affect, Urges and Smoking. PhD dissertation (unpublished), University of Washington, Seattle, WA, 2008.

61. Brown RA, Palm KM, Strong DR, Lejuez CW, Kahler CW, Zvolensky MJ, Hayes SC, Wilson KG, Gifford EV. Distress tolerance treatment for early-lapse smokers: rationale, program description, and preliminary findings. *Behav Modif*. 2008;32:302–332.

62. Hayes SC, Luoma JB, Bond FW, Masuda A, Lillis J. Acceptance and commitment therapy: model, processes and outcomes. *Behav Res Ther*. 2006;44:1–25.

63. Beck AT, Rush AJ, Shaw BF, Emery G. *Cognitive Therapy of Depression*. New York: Guilford Press; 1979.

64. Ma SH, Teasdale JD. Mindfulness-based cognitive therapy for depression: replication and exploration of differential relapse prevention effects. *J Consult Clin Psychol*. 2004;72:31–40.

65. Teasdale JD, Segal ZV, Williams JM, Ridgeway VA, Soulsby JM, Lau MA. Prevention of relapse/recurrence in major depression by mindfulness-based cognitive therapy. *J Consult Clin Psychol*. 2000;68:615–623.

66. Kenny MA, Williams JM. Treatment-resistant depressed patients show a good response to Mindfulness-Based Cognitive Therapy. *Behav Res Ther*. 2007;45:617–625.

67. Evans S, Ferrando S, Findler M, Stowell C, Smart C, Haglin D. Mindfulness-based cognitive therapy for generalized anxiety disorder. *J Anxiety Disord*. 2008;22(4):716–721. Epub 2007 July 22.

68. Carroll KM. Relapse prevention as a psychosocial treatment: a review of controlled clinical trials. *Exp Clin Psychopharmacol*. 1996;4:46–54.

69. Marlatt GA [Principal Investigator]. Efficacy of Mindfulness-Based Relapse Prevention. National Institute of Drug Abuse, Grant 1R21DA0119562, Years 2006–2008, University of Washington, Seattle.

70. Linehan MM, Armstrong HE, Suarez A, Allmon D, Heard HL. Cognitive-behavioral treatment of chronically parasuicidal borderline patients. *Arch Gen Psychiatry*. 1991;48:1060–1064.

71. Linehan MM, Dimeff LA. *Dialectical Behavior Therapy for Substance Abuse Treatment Manual*. Seattle, WA: University of Seattle; 1997.

72. Marcus MT [Principal Investigator]. Stress Reduction in Therapeutic Community Treatment. National Institute of Drug Abuse, Grant 5R01DA017719, Years 2004–2008, University of Texas, Houston.

73. Ernst E, Pittler MH, Stevinson C, White A. Ramdomised clinical trials: pragmatic or fastidious? *Focus Alt Compl Ther*. 2001;63:179–180.

74. Davidson RJ, Kabat-Zinn J, Schumacher J, Rosenkranz M, Muller D, Santorelli SF, Urbanowski F, Harrington A, Bonus K, Sheridan JF. Alterations in brain and immune function produced by mindfulness meditation. *Psychosom Med*. 2003;65:564–570.

75. Grossman P, Niemann L, Schmidt S, Walach H. Mindfulness-based stress reduction and health benefits. A meta-analysis. *J Psychosom Res*. 2004;57:35–43.

76. Praissman S. Mindfulness-based stress reduction: a literature review and clinician's guide. *J Am Acad Nurse Pract*. 2008;20:212–6.

77. Tang YY, Ma Y, Wang J, Fan Y, Feng S, Lu Q, Yu Q, Sui D, Rothbart MK, Fan M, Posner MI. Short-term

meditation training improves attention and self-regulation. *Proc Natl Acad Sci USA.* 2007;104:17152–17156.

78. Ciraulo DA, Piechniczek-Buczek J, Iscan EN. Outcome predictors in substance use disorders. *Psychiatr Clin North Am.* 2003;26:381–409.

79. Fox HC, Bergquist KL, Hong KI, Sinha R. Stress-induced and alcohol cue-induced craving in recently abstinent alcohol-dependent individuals. *Alcohol Clin Exp Res.* 2007;31:395–403.

80. Kazdin AE. Methodology, design, and evaluation of in psychotherapy research. In: Bergin AE, Garfield SL, eds. *Handbook of Psychotherapy and Behavior Change.* New York: Wiley; 1994:19–71.

81. Project MATCH Research Group. Matching Alcoholism Treatments to Client Heterogeneity: Project MATCH posttreatment drinking outcomes. *J Stud Alcohol.* 1997;58:7–29.

82. Anton RF, O'Malley SS, Ciraulo DA, Cisler RA, Couper D, Donovan DM, Gastfriend DR, Hosking JD, Johnson BA, LoCastro JS, Longabaugh R, Mason BJ, Mattson ME, Miller WR, Pettinati HM, Randall CL, Swift R, Weiss RD, Williams LD, Zweben, A; COMBINE study Research Group. Combined pharmacotherapies and behavioral interventions for alcohol dependence: the COMBINE study: a randomized controlled trial. *JAMA.* 2006;295:2003–2017.

83. Marlatt GA. Buddhist philosophy and the treatment of addictive behavior. *Cogn Behav Pract.* 2002;9:44–50.

84. Smith BW, Shelley BM, Dalen J, Wiggins K, Tooley E, Bernard J. A pilot study comparing the effects of mindfulness-based and cognitive-behavioral stress reduction. *J Altern Complement Med.* 2008;14:251–258.

85. Zautra AJ, Davis MC, Reich JW, Nicassario P, Tennen H, Finan P, Kratz A, Parrish B, Irwin MR. Comparison of cognitive behavioral and mindfulness meditation interventions on adaptation to rheumatoid arthritis for patients with and without history of recurrent depression. *J Consult Clin Psychol.* 2008;76:408–421.

86. Teasdale JD, Segal ZV, Williams JM. Mindfulness training and problem formulation. *Clin Psychol Sci Pr.* 2003;10:157–160.

87. Marcus MT, Liehr PR, Schmitz J, Moeller FG, Swank P, Fine M, Cron S, Granmayeh LK, Carroll DD. Behavioral therapies trials: a case example. *Nurs Res.* 2007;56:210–216.

Mindfulness-Based Relapse Prevention for Substance Use Disorders: A Pilot Efficacy Trial

Sarah Bowen, PhD
Neharika Chawla, MS
Susan E. Collins, PhD
Katie Witkiewitz, PhD
Sharon Hsu, BA
Joel Grow, BA
Seema Clifasefi, PhD
Michelle Garner, PhD
Anne Douglass, BA
Mary E. Larimer, PhD
Alan Marlatt, PhD

ABSTRACT. The current study is the first randomized-controlled trial evaluating the feasibility and initial efficacy of an 8-week outpatient Mindfulness-Based Relapse Prevention (MBRP) program as compared to treatment as usual (TAU). Participants were 168 adults with substance use disorders who had recently completed intensive inpatient or outpatient treatment. Assessments were administered pre-intervention, post-intervention, and 2 and 4 months post-intervention. Feasibility of MBRP was demonstrated by consistent homework compliance, attendance, and participant satisfaction. Initial efficacy was supported by significantly lower rates of substance use in those who received MBRP as compared to those in TAU over the 4-month post-intervention period. Additionally, MBRP participants demonstrated greater decreases in craving, and increases in acceptance and acting with awareness as compared to TAU. Results from this initial trial support the feasibility and initial efficacy of MBRP as an aftercare approach for individuals who have recently completed an intensive treatment for substance use disorders.

Sarah Bowen, Neharika Chawla, Susan E. Collins, Sharon Hsu, Joel Grow, Seema Clifasefi, Anne Douglass, and Alan Marlatt are affiliated with the Addictive Behaviors Research Center, Department of Psychology, University of Washington, Seattle, Washington, USA.

Katie Witkiewitz is affiliated with the Alcohol and Drug Abuse Institute, University of Washington, Seattle, Washington, USA.

Michelle Garner is affiliated with the School of Social Work, University of Washington, Tacoma, Washington, USA.

Mary E. Larimer is affiliated with the Department of Psychiatry and Behavioral Sciences, University of Washington, Seattle, Washington, USA.

This research was supported by National Institute on Drug Abuse grant R21 DA010562.

INTRODUCTION

With rates of relapse following substance abuse treatment estimated at over 60% (1), substance use disorders are often described as "chronic relapsing conditions" (2,3). The most commonly available treatments in many developed countries are 12-step or mutual support groups (4). Participation in12-step programs is associated with greater abstinence (5); however, these approaches may not be clinically indicated for individuals adverse to the disease model of addiction (6) or whose spiritual beliefs and/or lifestyle are in conflict with the 12-step philosophy. As an alternative to 12-step programs, Relapse Prevention (RP) (7), a cognitive-behavioral treatment, focuses on responses to high-risk situations, combining skills-training with cognitive interventions to prevent or limit relapse. RP has been disseminated for treatment of several types of substance abuse (8–12) with considerable empirical support (13–20). Although RP suggests promising advancement in treatment, relapse remains a significant problem for 44% to 70% of clients (21). Integration of further efficacious treatment components may enhance RP treatment effects (18).

Mindfulness has been described as "paying attention in a particular way: on purpose, in the present moment, and non-judgmentally" (22). Many therapeutic orientations, such as Mindfulness-Based Stress Reduction (MBSR) (23) and Mindfulness-Based Cognitive Therapy for depression (MBCT) (24), use mindfulness techniques and practices, leading to growing evidence of its benefits (24–30). Research on mindfulness in the treatment of substance use disorders is beginning to receive attention in scientific literature (31–33). Theoretical foundations for integration of mindfulness with traditional cognitive-behavioral relapse prevention (34) suggest that mindfulness may help develop a detached and de-centered relationship to thoughts and feelings, preventing escalation of thought patterns that may lead to relapse (35,36). Via increased awareness, regulation, and tolerance of potential precipitants of relapse, mindfulness may enhance ability to cope with relapse triggers, interrupting the previous cycle of automatic substance use behavior. In the event of a lapse, awareness and acceptance fostered by mindfulness may aid in recognition and minimization of the blame, guilt, and negative thinking that increase risk of relapse (37).

Mindfulness-Based Relapse Prevention (MBRP), a novel mindfulness-based aftercare approach, integrates core aspects of RP with practices adapted from MBSR (23) and MBCT (24). Identification of high-risk situations remains central to the treatment. Participants are trained to recognize early warning signs for relapse, increase awareness of internal (i.e., emotional and cognitive) and external (i.e., situational) cues previously associated with substance use, develop effective coping skills, and enhance self-efficacy. Mindfulness practices included in MBRP are intended to raise awareness of triggers, monitor internal reactions, and foster more skillful behavioral choices. The practices focus on increasing acceptance and tolerance of positive and negative physical, emotional, and cognitive states, such as craving, thereby decreasing the need to alleviate associated discomfort by engaging in substance use.

The current pilot randomized controlled trial (RCT) evaluated the feasibility and initial efficacy of MBRP in comparison to treatment as usual (TAU) among individuals with substance use disorders. The study assessed treatment effects on substance use outcomes as well as key secondary processes including craving, mindfulness, and acceptance. It was hypothesized that participation in MBRP would be associated with greater reductions in substance use, and greater increases in mindfulness and acceptance in MBRP versus TAU participants.

METHODS

Participants

Participants ($N = 168$) were recruited from a private, nonprofit agency providing a continuum of care for alcohol and drug use disorders, serving approximately 126 clients per month in both inpatient and outpatient settings. Approximately 57% of the agency's outpatient and 2% of inpatient clients are legally mandated to substance abuse treatment, and 19% of outpatient and 75% of inpatient clients are homeless. Roughly 55% of clients complete treatment as recommended.

Eligible participants were between the ages of 18 and 70, fluent in English, had completed intensive outpatient or inpatient treatment in the previous 2 weeks, and were medically cleared for participation. Exclusion criteria included psychosis, dementia, imminent suicide risk, significant withdrawal risk, or need for more intensive treatment.

Measures

With the exception of demographics questions, administered at baseline, the same battery of measures was administered at baseline, immediately following the 8-week intervention period, and 2 and 4 months post-intervention. All assessments were completed onsite via an Internet-based assessment program, with study staff available to guide participants through assessment procedures.

Eligibility Screening

Eligibility was determined via telephone assessment. The "Psychotic and Associated Symptoms" sections of the Structured Clinical Interview for DSM-IV, Axis I (SCID-I) (38) assessed lifetime experience of a psychotic disorder. The SCID-I has demonstrated reliability and validity in such settings. Suicidality was assessed using the suicide section of the Hamilton Depression Inventory (39), and a single item from the Brief Symptom Inventory (40) ("How much were you distressed by thoughts of ending your life?").

Substance Use

The Timeline Followback (TLFB) (41) assessed daily use of alcohol (using a standard drink conversion chart) and drugs. At baseline, participants were asked to report for the 60 days prior to initial inpatient or outpatient treatment admission. For all other assessments, participants reported on the 60 days immediately prior to assessment. The TLFB has demonstrated good reliability and validity with both online and in-person administration (42).

Alcohol and Drug Craving

The Penn Alcohol Craving Scale (PACS) (43) was adapted to include both alcohol and drug craving. The PACS is a 5-item, self-report measure assessing frequency, intensity, and duration of craving, and overall rating of craving for the previous week. It has shown excellent internal consistency and predictive validity for alcohol relapse. Its internal consistency in the current sample was .87.

Alcohol and Drug Use Consequences

The 15-item Short Inventory of Problems (SIP-AD) (44), adapted from the Inventory of Drug Use Consequences-2R (InDUC-2R) (45), assessed impulse control, social responsibility, and physical, interpersonal, and intrapersonal consequences. The correlation between InDUC and SIP-AD has been shown to be strong ($r = .96$) (44), and internal consistency in the current study was .96.

Mindfulness

The Five Factor Mindfulness Questionnaire (FFMQ) consisting of 39 items rated on a 5-point Likert scale, assessed 5 factors of mindfulness (46). The FFMQ has demonstrated good internal consistency (46). Internal consistency in the current study was .91, with subscale alphas ranging from .80 to .87.

Acceptance

The Acceptance and Action Questionnaire (AAQ) (47) is a 9-item instrument assessing acceptance versus avoidance and control of negative private experiences. Items are rated on a 7-point Likert-type scale, with higher scores indicating greater acceptance. Lower scores have been associated with increased levels of psychopathology and decreased quality of life (48). Its internal consistency in the current study was .68.

Meditation Practice

MBRP participants recorded the type and number of minutes of mindfulness practice using a worksheet submitted weekly throughout the intervention. In addition, average days per week and minutes per meditation session were assessed at all time points.

Participant Feedback

Participants attending the final MBRP session completed a questionnaire assessing course satisfaction on a 10-point Likert scale ranging from "Not at all"' to "Very." Questions included "How important has this program been to you?" and "How likely are you to continue engaging in formal mindfulness practice after this course?"

Treatment

MBRP

The treatment was delivered in 8 weekly, 2-hour group sessions, following the protocol outlined in the MBRP treatment manual (Bowen, Chawla, and Marlatt, 48a). Each group (6 to 10 participants) was facilitated by 2 therapists. Each session had a central theme, with meditation practices and related RP discussions and exercises. Themes included "automatic-pilot" and its relationship to relapse, recognizing thoughts and emotions in relation to triggers, integrating mindfulness practices into daily life, practicing the skills in high-risk situations, and the role of thoughts in relapse.

Sessions began with a 20- to 30-minute guided meditation and involved a variety of experiential exercises, interspersed with discussions of the role of mindfulness in relapse prevention and review of homework assignments. Participants were assigned daily exercises to practice between sessions, and were provided with meditation CDs (49) for practice outside group sessions.

TAU

Participants in the TAU condition remained in standard outpatient aftercare provided by the treatment agency, designed to maintain abstinence through a 12-step, process-oriented format. Several groups were offered as part of TAU, with a weekly aftercare groups serving as the primary and regularly attended component. Topics included rational thinking skills (50), grief and loss, assertiveness, self-esteem, goal setting,

effects of alcohol and other drugs on interpersonal relations and experience, and related themes. RP skills, based upon the disease model of addiction (51), were included in some of the groups. TAU groups lasted approximately 1.5 hours, and met 1 to 2 times weekly depending on client need, as compared to the 2-hour weekly MBRP group sessions. TAU groups were not regularly assigned homework.

Therapists

Therapists facilitating MBRP groups held master's degrees in psychology or social work, and were experienced in delivery of cognitive-behavioral interventions. Several had extensive backgrounds in mindfulness meditation. Therapists participated in several weeks of intensive training, engaged in daily meditation practice, and received weekly supervision throughout the trial from therapists experienced in mindfulness-based treatments. Therapists facilitating the TAU groups were licensed Chemical Dependency Counselors, with varying levels of experience in the delivery of outpatient aftercare services.

Design and Procedure

All study procedures were approved by the University of Washington Institutional Review Board. Participants were recruited near the end of their inpatient or outpatient substance abuse treatment through flyers and referrals from agency or research staff. Potential participants contacted research staff by telephone, were verbally consented for screening, and completed a 30- to 45-minute telephone eligibility screen.

Following informed consent procedures, eligible participants completed an on-site baseline assessment, with research staff available to assist or answer questions. Following completion of the assessment, participants were randomly assigned, using a computerized random number generator, to either 8 weeks of MBRP or continuation of their existing TAU. Those refusing randomization were given community treatment resource information. Participants randomized to MBRP agreed to discontinue TAU for the 8 weeks of the MBRP course duration, and to resume TAU following completion of MBRP. TAU participants were given the opportunity to attend the MBRP course free of charge upon completion of their 4-month post-intervention assessment.

Participants who did not complete their scheduled follow-up assessments were contacted via telephone to document their substance use. All participants received $45 gift cards for completion of both baseline and post-intervention assessments, and $50 gift cards for each post-intervention assessment. All participants were encouraged to continue attending 12-step or other self-help groups as recommended by the treatment agency.

Statistical Analysis

Variables were examined for univariate outliers and deviation from expected distributions. The substance-use variables were positively skewed count variables. The AAQ and the FFMQ were continuous, normally distributed variables. The PACS was a positively skewed, continuous variable that fit the gamma distribution. Examination of postestimation residual plots indicated no extreme outliers. Chi-square and t tests were used to examine baseline treatment group differences at baseline.

Population-averaged generalized estimating equations (52) were conducted to test treatment effects on substance-use and process outcomes using STATA-10 statistical program (53). Poisson distributions were specified for the positively skewed substance-use outcomes (54). To enhance interpretability, the log link was used for these models, and coefficients were exponentiated to yield incident rate ratios (IRRs). For analyses involving alcohol or drug (AOD) days, the natural log of the days of valid self-report data was entered as an offset variable. Normal or gamma distributions were used for analyses involving the process variables. To accommodate the longitudinal and incomplete data, an exchangeable correlation structure was used, and bootstrapping was applied to correct standard errors (55). The count, integer, or continuous nature of the outcome variables precluded the use of intent-to-treat analyses; however, recent simulation studies have shown that the estimation method employed in this study (i.e., maximum

likelihood estimation) is less biased and more precise in dealing with missing data than traditional data imputation methods, such as assuming use for missing observations (intent-to-treat methods) or carrying the last observation forward (56).

Models included 6 predictors: a linear time (t) variable that modeled linear change in the variables from baseline, post-intervention, and 2- and 4-month post-intervention (coded as 0, 1, 2 and 3, respectively); a quadratic time (t^2) variable; dummy-coded treatment effects (1 = MBRP, 0 = TAU); and t and $t^2 \times$ treatment interactions. The 2-tailed alpha level was $P = .05$ for all analyses. Results are presented as mean (standard deviation [SD]) unless otherwise specified.

RESULTS

Of screened participants ($N = 260$), 187 met eligibility criteria. Nine declined participation, 9 failed to complete the baseline assessment, and 1 refused randomization, reducing the overall sample to 168.

The majority of the final sample (63.7%) was male, with an average age of 40. 5 (10.3) years. Approximately half identified as Caucasian (51.8%), followed by African American (28.6%), Multiracial (15.3%), and Native American (7.7%). The majority had at least a high-school diploma (71.6%). Approximately 41.3% was unemployed and 32.9% reported receiving some form of public assistance. The majority (62.3%) earned less than $4999 per year. Primary substances of abuse were alcohol (45.2%), cocaine/crack (36.2%), methamphetamines (13.7%), opiates/heroin (7.1%), marijuana (5.4%), and other (1.9%). Approximately 19.1% reported polysubstance use.

Treatment Group Differences at Baseline

Racial distribution differed between groups at baseline (χ^2 (1, $N = 168) = 5.51$, $P = .02$); the MBRP group consisted of a higher proportion of White participants (63%) than TAU (45%). This difference was a nonsystematic effect of randomization, and there were no differences in attrition between White and non-White participants in the MBRP group (χ^2 (1, $N = 93$) = .631, $P = .43$). To control for this baseline difference, race was used as a covariate in all analyses. There were no other baseline treatment differences on demographic or main outcome variables (all $P > .14$). Other sociodemographic variables, including gender, ethnicity, and severity of initial substance use, were examined in primary analyses as potential covariates and moderators of the treatment effects. None were significant (all $P > .05$), and they were not included in final models.

Treatment Compliance, Attrition, and Satisfaction

Approximately 61%, 57%, and 73% of the sample ($N = 168$) completed post-intervention and 2-month and 4-month follow-up assessments, respectively. Attrition did not significantly differ between groups at any time point and the predictors in each model were not significantly associated with missing data on dependent variables.

MBRP participants reported attending 5.2 (2.4) or 65% of treatment sessions. Attendance rates in TAU groups were not available; however, a significant difference was noted between the MBRP (12.8 ± 4.9) and TAU (9.8 ± 8.2) groups in number of treatment hours received during the 8-week intervention period (Mann-Whitney U test, $U = 2113.5$, $P < .001$). Total number of treatment hours was therefore used as a covariate in all primary analyses.

Most MBRP participants (86%) reported practicing meditation post-intervention, and 54% reported continued practice at 4 months post-intervention for an average of 4.7 ± 4.0 days/week and 29.9 ± 19.5 minutes per session. On a 10-point Likert scale, participants rated the MBRP course as highly important (8.3 ± 1.4) and reported a high likelihood of continuing formal (8.9 ± 1.2) and informal (8.9 ± 1.7) meditation practices.

Primary Outcomes

The AOD use model was statistically significant (Wald χ^2 (7, $N = 163$) = 97.72, $P < .001$). (See Table 1 for means.) As shown in Table 2,

TABLE 1. Means (Standard Deviations) for Alcohol and Other Drug Use and Process Variables During the Study

Variables	Baseline		Posttest		2 months post-intervention		4 months post-intervention	
	MBRP	TAU	MBRP	TAU	MBRP	TAU	MBRP	TAU
AOD days	27.0	28.9	.1	2.6	2.1	5.4	5.1	5.1
	(24.0)	(24.8)	(.3)	(9.1)	(7.2)	(14.7)	(14.9)	(15.3)
	(n = 93)	(n = 70)	(n = 77)	(n = 56)	(n = 74)	(n = 56)	(n = 69)	(n = 49)
SIP	11.1	11.7	2.3	3.4	2.9	3.8	3.1	3.9
	(5.4)	(4.7)	(4.5)	(5.6)	(5.3)	(5.8)	(5.4)	(5.8)
	(n = 93)	(n = 75)	(n = 62)	(n = 42)	(n = 53)	(n = 42)	(n = 71)	(n = 52)
PACS	1.6	1.7	1.1	1.7	1.0	1.4	1.1	1.3
	(1.1)	(1.4)	(1.1)	(1.4)	(1.0)	(1.5)	(1.3)	(1.5)
	(n = 91)	(n = 75)	(n = 62)	(n = 41)	(n = 53)	(n = 42)	(n = 70)	(n = 52)
AAQ	47.1	47.2	51.2	47.6	49.6	48.8	50.2	50.3
	(7.5)	(9.6)	(7.8)	(10.0)	(9.1)	(9.6)	(7.5)	(10.3)
	(n = 76)	(n = 72)	(n = 56)	(n = 40)	(n = 51)	(n = 39)	(n = 63)	(n = 50)
FFMQ-ACT	26.2	27.7	27.1	26.5	27.9	25.3	26.2	28.8
	(6.2)	(6.9)	(7.0)	(7.2)	(6.3)	(7.2)	(5.8)	(7.9)
	(n = 84)	(n = 72)	(n = 55)	(n = 40)	(n = 52)	(n = 37)	(n = 61)	(n = 48)

Note. MBRP = Mindfulness-Based Relapse Prevention; TAU = treatment as usual; AOD = alcohol and other drug use; SIP = Short Inventory of Problems; PACS = Penn Alcohol Craving Scale; AAQ = Acceptance and Action Questionnaire; FFMQ-ACT = Five-Factor Mindfulness Questionnaire–Act With Awareness Scale.

TABLE 2. Generalized Estimating Equations Models Evaluating Treatment Effects on Main and Process Outcomes

Predictors	AOD use ($N = 163$)			
	IRR	CI (95%)	z	P
t	.10	.05–.24	−5.31	<.001
t^2	1.80	1.42–2.27	4.86	<.001
Total treatment hrs	1.00	.97–1.03	−.04	.97
Race	1.02	.76–1.36	.10	.92
Treatment	.92	.67–1.25	−.54	.59
t × treatment	.14	.03–.70	−2.40	.02
t^2 × treatment	1.91	1.16–3.15	2.55	.01
Predictors	Craving ($N = 166$)			
	Exp(B)	CI (95%)	z	P
t	1.06	.76–1.47	.35	.73
t^2	.95	.86–1.07	−.83	.41
Total treatment hours	.99	.97–1.01	−1.34	.18
Race	1.55	1.24–1.94	3.84	<.001
Treatment	.84	.66–1.06	−1.46	.14
t × treatment	.68	.49–.95	−2.27	.02
t^2 × treatment	1.13	1.01–1.26	2.21	.03
Predictors	Acceptance ($N = 163$)			
	β	CI (95%)	z	P
t	.03	−.26, .32	0.21	.84
t^2	.06	−.25, .36	0.36	.72
Total treatment hours	−.05	−.18, .08	−.71	.48
Race	−.05	−.21, .10	−0.68	.50
Treatment	.03	−.14, .20	0.35	.73
t × treatment	.44	.01, .87	2.00	.045
t^2 × treatment	−.40	−.80, −.01	−1.98	.047
Predictors	Acting with awareness ($N = 165$)			
	β	CI (95%)	z	P
t	−.48	−.85, −.11	−2.53	.01
t^2	.52	.10, .93	2.44	.02
Total treatment hours	−.03	−.20, .13	−0.40	.69
Race	−.09	−.23, .06	−1.18	.24
Treatment	−.09	−.27, .09	−1.03	.30
t × treatment	.67	.15, 1.18	2.54	.01
t^2 × treatment	−.61	−1.11, −.11	−2.43	.02

Note. For all models: t = linear time predictor (0 = baseline; 1 = posttest; 2 = 2-month follow-up; 3 = 4-month follow-up); t^2 = quadratic time predictor. IRR = incident rate ratio or the rate of increase/decrease outcome variable based on a one-unit change in the predictor, where IRR values greater than 1 indicate rate increases, and values less than 1 indicate rate decreases. Exp(B) = exponentiated gamma-log coefficient (values less than 1 represent inverse associations; values greater than 1 represent positive associations). β = standardized regression coefficient (negative values represent inverse associations; positive values represent positive associations). SE = bootstrapped standard error. CI (95%) = 95% confidence intervals. The treatment variable was dummy coded with MBRP treatment group = 1, TAU = 0. Self-reported race was dummy coded with 1 = White, 0 = non-White.

For alcohol and other drug use (AOD) model: An additional series of post hoc, cross-sectional, Poisson regressions tested treatment differences at each time point. The MBRP group reported significantly lower AOD use at both post-intervention (IRR = .02, P < .001) and 2 months post-intervention (IRR = .39, P < .001); however, this difference was reduced to nonsignificant at 4 months post-intervention (IRR = 1.11, P = .21).

t and t^2 were significant predictors of AOD use days following the intervention. The significant main effects for t were qualified by a significant t × Treatment interaction, which indicated that AOD use decreased to a greater extent among MBRP versus TAU participants. Specifically, the MBRP group showed an average 86% decrease in AOD use for each 2-month increase in linear time. Two months post-intervention, MBRP participants reported an average of 2.1 days of use, and TAU participants reported an average of 5.4 days (see Table 2). The significant t^2 × Treatment interaction also indicated a curvilinear effect of treatment on AOD use, which suggested that the treatment gains made by MBRP participants, compared to TAU participants, decayed by 4 months post-intervention.

The omnibus model for substance-use problems (Wald χ^2 (7, $N = 163$) = 135.14, $P < .001$) was significant. Significant main effects for t (IRR = .25, $P < .001$) and t^2 (IRR = 1.44, $P = .001$) indicated that, overall, participants showed a curvilinear decrease in experience of substance-use problems over time. There were no significant treatment interactions or main effects of treatment on substance use problems ($P > .68$).

Process Outcomes

The craving (PACS) model was statistically significant (Wald χ^2 (7, $N = 166$) = 37.60, $P < .001$). As shown in Table 2, race was a significant covariate: overall White participants showed higher craving than non-White participants. Secondary analyses, however, showed that race did not interact with time or treatment to have an effect on craving ($P > .05$). The significant t × Treatment interaction shown in Table 2 indicated that, over time, craving decreased to a greater extent among MBRP versus TAU participants. The significant t^2 × Treatment interaction suggests the magnitude of decreases in craving among MBRP participants plateaued over the 4-month post-intervention period.

The acceptance (AAQ) model was statistically significant (Wald χ^2 (7, $N = 163$) = 16.25, $P = .02$). There was a significant t × Treatment interaction such that, over time, acceptance increased more among MBRP participants than among TAU participants (see Table 2). The significant $t^2 \times$ treatment interaction showed that increases in acceptance among MBRP participants plateaued over 4 months post-intervention.

The acting with awareness (FFMQ-ACT) model was marginally significant (Wald χ^2 (7, $N = 165) = 13.03$, $P = .07$). As shown in Table 2, t and t^2 were significant predictors of acting with awareness. The significant main effects for t were qualified by a significant t $\times$ Treatment interaction, suggesting that acting with awareness increased to a greater extent among MBRP versus TAU participants, for whom it decreased. At 4 months post-intervention, however, the significant $t^2 \times$ treatment interaction showed that increases in acting with awareness among MBRP participants plateaued. Models for the other subscales of the FFMQ evinced nonsignificant treatment effects or omnibus model tests ($P > .05$).

No side effects of treatment or adverse events during the course of the study were detected or reported.

DISCUSSION

Results of the current study provide evidence for the feasibility and initial efficacy of MBRP, offering empirical support for MBRP as an alternative to standard-of-care 12-step-based or related aftercare programs. Outcomes suggest significant improvement in MBRP versus TAU participants in days of substance use, craving, awareness, and acceptance. Differences were not evident on other aspects of mindfulness (observing, describing, nonjudgment of inner experience, and nonreactivity to inner experience). Additionally, although participants in both groups reported a decrease in substance-related problems, decreases were not significantly different between groups. Finally, analyses of sociodemographic variables (gender, ethnicity, and severity of initial substance use) did not show evidence of their moderating effects on treatment outcomes.

Good participant compliance, reflected in attendance and continued meditation practice, supports feasibility of MBRP. Over half of the sample continued formal meditation practice for at least 4 months post-intervention, supporting acceptability of MBRP in this population. Positive course ratings and the absence of significant differences in attrition rates between the MBRP and TAU arms indicate tolerability of and interest in MBRP among participants with substance use disorders. The MBRP intervention appears safe as indicated by lack of reported side effects or adverse events.

Significant decreases were found in overall days of substance use post-intervention among participants in MBRP versus those in TAU group. These gains appeared to diminish at 4 months post-intervention, however, with those in MBRP returning to levels similar to those in TAU. This reduction in treatment effects over time may be attributed to the study design, which entailed MBRP participants returning to TAU groups following their 8-week MBRP course. The TAU groups did not necessarily foster continuation of practices and perspectives learned in MBRP. It is therefore not surprising that MBRP treatment gains were not fully maintained. These findings suggest need for continued support and maintenance following MBRP treatment. Future studies may benefit from inclusion of continuing, intervention-consistent support, which has been found to improve treatment efficacy in substance use disorders (57,58).

In view of MBRP's focus on increasing awareness, decreasing judgment, and shifting from "reacting" to "skillful responding" (all key "descriptors" of mindfulness) absence of significant differences in FFMQ factors representing observing, describing, nonjudgment, and nonreactivity is surprising. However, evidence of processes targeted by MBRP is reflected in differential increases in acceptance and acting with awareness, and decreases in craving. A substantial body of literature documents harmful effects of suppression or avoidance of cognitive and affective responses on a variety of psychological and health outcomes (59–63). A central focus of MBRP is thus to increase awareness and acceptance of physical, emotional, and cognitive states. Increases in acceptance and acting with awareness, reflected in the current study, may indicate a decreased need to alleviate discomfort with substance use, and an increase in intentional versus reactive behavior.

Reductions in severity of craving in the current study may be explained by increases in awareness of sensations, thoughts, and emotions that accompany craving, coupled with encouraging acceptance of and nonreactivity to the craving response. Repeated exposure to triggering stimuli during which participants practice non-reactivity may, over time, result in habituation, thereby decreasing the intensity of the initial craving reaction (64).

Taken together, results from the current study are consistent with the underlying rationale for mindfulness-based treatments, designed to interrupt reactive behaviors and encourage skillful responses to challenging situations (23,26). Further, results are consistent with neurobiological research indicating associations between mindfulness practice and changes in brain regions involved in modulation of arousal and emotion regulation (65,66).

The current study has several strengths. To our knowledge, this is the first RCT evaluating the efficacy of a mindfulness-based intervention for substance use disorders and the prevention of relapse. The study provides preliminary support for feasibility, acceptability, and efficacy of mindfulness-based therapies for substance use disorders in an ethnically diverse and challenging population, with high rates of homelessness and involvement with the legal system. Although other acceptance- and mindfulness-based treatments or protocols with related components have been applied to substance abuse samples, MBRP is uniquely designed to address the specific needs of this population.

The current study also has several limitations. The brevity of the follow-up period restricted the ability to examine effects of MBRP on long-term outcomes. Although research indicates up to two thirds of individuals relapse within the first 3 months following treatment (21), rates of substance use remained low in both groups throughout the study, limiting variability and thus power to find significant between-group differences. Although retrospective self-report of substance use using may present another potential limitation, the TLFB method is considered a gold standard of substance use assessment. However, additional methods, such as urine toxicology testing, would strengthen the validity of these reports. Finally, due to attrition, complete data were not available for all participants during the follow-up period. Although attrition in the current study is comparable to studies in similar populations (67), conclusions that can be drawn about treatment effects for the complete sample are limited.

In conclusion, this RCT demonstrates empirical promise for feasibility and initial efficacy of MBRP as an aftercare treatment for substance use disorders, and provides preliminary support for the theoretical framework behind mindfulness meditation as a therapy for addictive behaviors. In the tradition of well-established MBSR (28) and MBCT (26) programs, MBRP extends the populations for which mindfulness meditation therapies can be used to alleviate distress and foster fundamental change in maladaptive patterns of behavior.

REFERENCES

1. McLellan AT, Lewis DC, O'Brien CP, Kleber HD. Drug dependence, a chronic mental illness: implications for treatment, insurance, and outcomes evaluation. *JAMA.* 2000;284:1689–1695.

2. Connors GJ, Maisto SA, Donovan DM. Conceptualizations of relapse: a summary of psychological and psychobiological models. *Addiction* 1996; 91:5–13.

3. Dixon L, McNary S, Lehman AF. Remission of substance use disorder among psychiatric inpatients with mental illness. *Am J Psychiatry* 1998; 155:239–243.

4. Room R. Mutual help movements for alcohol problems: an international perspective. *Addict Res.* 1998; 6:131–145.

5. Tonigan JS, Toscova R, Miller WR. Meta-analysis of the literature on Alcoholics Anonymous: sample and study characteristics moderate findings. *J Stud Alcohol.* 1996; 57:65–72.

6. Marlatt GA, Witkiewitz K. Harm reduction approaches to alcohol use: health promotion, prevention, and treatment. *Addict Behav.* 2002; 27:867–886.

7. Marlatt GA, Gordon JR, eds. *Relapse Prevention: Maintenance Strategies in the Treatment of Addictive Behaviors.* New York: Guilford Press; 1985.

8. Baker A, Boggs TG, Lewin TJ. Randomized controlled trial of brief cognitive-behavioural interventions among regular users of amphetamine. Addiction 2001 96:1279–1287.

9. Carroll KM. Treating drug dependence: recent advances and old truths. In: Miller WR, Heather N, eds. *Treating Addictive Behaviors.* 2nd ed. Applied Clinical Psychology; New York: Plenum Press; 1998:217–229.

10. Kosten TR. Buprenorphine for opioid detoxification: a brief review. *Addict Disord Treat.* 2003; 2:107–112.

11. Roffman RA, Stephens RS, Simpson EE, Whitaker DL. Treatment of marijuana dependence: preliminary results. *J Psychoactive Drugs.* 1990; 20:129–137.

12. Schmitz JM., Stotts AL, Rhoades HM, Grabowski J. Naltrexone and relapse prevention treatment for cocaine-dependent patients. *Addict Behav.* 2001; 26:167–180.

13. Carroll KM. Relapse prevention as a psychosocial treatment: a review of controlled clinical trials. *Exp Clin Psychopharmacol.* 1996; 4:46–54.

14. Kadden RM. Behavioral and cognitive-behavioral treatment for alcoholism research opportunities. *Addict Behav.* 2001; 26:489–507.

15. Monti PM, Rohsenow DJ, Michalec E, Martin RA, Abrams DB. Brief coping skills treatment for cocaine abuse: substance use outcomes at three months. *Addiction.* 1997; 92:1717–1728.

16. Fals-Stewart W, O'Farrell TJ. Behavioral family counseling and naltrexone for male opioid dependent patients. *J Consult Clin Psychol.* 2003; 71: 432–442.

17. Bien TH, Miller WR, Tonigan JS. Brief interventions for alcohol problems: a review. *Addiction* 1993; 88: 315–335.

18. Irvin JE, Bowers CA, Dunn ME, Wang MC. Efficacy of relapse prevention: a meta-analytic review. *J Consult Clin Psychol.* 1999; 67: 563–570.

19. Carroll KM, Rounsaville BJ, Gawin FH. A comparative trial of psychotherapies for ambulatory cocaine abusers: relapse prevention and interpersonal psychotherapy. *Am J Drug Alcohol Abuse.* 1991; 17:229–247.

20. Davis JR, Glaros AG. Relapse prevention and smoking cessation. *Addict Behav.* 1986; 11: 105–114.

21. Pickens R, Hatsukami D, Spicer J, Svikis D. Relapse by alcohol abusers. *Alcohol Clin Exp Res.* 1985; 9:244–247.

22. Kabat-Zinn J. *Wherever You Go, There You Are: Mindfulness Meditation in Everyday Life.* New York: Hyperion; 1994.

23. Kabat-Zinn J. Full *Catastrophe Living: Using the Wisdom of Your Body and Mind to Face Stress, Pain, and Illness.* New York: Delacorte; 1990.

24. Teasdale JD, Segal ZV, Williams JMG, Ridgeway VA, Soulsby JM, Lau MA. Prevention of relapse/recurrence in major depression by mindfulness-based cognitive therapy. *J Consult Clin Psychol.* 2000; 68:615–623.

25. Ma SH, Teasdale JD. Mindfulness-based cognitive therapy for depression: replication and exploration of differential relapse prevention effects. *J Consult Clin Psychol.* 2004; 72:31–40.

26. Segal ZV, Williams JMG, Teasdale JD. *Mindfulness-Based Cognitive Therapy for Depression: A New Approach to Preventing Relapse.* New York: Guilford Press; 2002.

27. Kristeller JL, Hallett CB. An exploratory study of an meditation-based intervention for binge eating disorder. *J Health Psychol.* 1999; 4:357–363.

28. Kabat-Zinn J, Massion A, Kristeller J, Peterson LG, Fletcher KE, Pbert L, Lenderking WR, Santorelli SF. Effectiveness of a meditation-based stress reduction intervention in the treatment of anxiety disorders. *Am J Psychiatry.* 1992; 149:936–943.

29. Goldenberg DL, Kaplan KH, Nadeau MG, Brodeur C, Smith S, Schmid CH. A controlled study of a stress-reduction, cognitive-behavioral treatment program in fibromyalgia. *J Muscoskel Pain.* 1994; 2:53–66.

30. Roth B, Creasor T. Mindfulness meditation-based stress reduction: experience with a bilingual inner-city program. *Nurse Pract.* 1997; 22:150–176.

31. Bowen S, Witkiewitz K, Dillworth T, Chawla N, Simpson T, Ostafin B, Larimer M, Blume A, Parks GA, Marlatt GA. Mindfulness meditation and substance use in an incarcerated population. *Psychol Addict Behav.* 2006; 20:343–347.

32. Davis J, Fleming M, Bonus K, Baker T. A pilot study on mindfulness based stress reduction for smokers. BMC Complement *Altern Med.* 2007; 7:2–2.

33. Zgierska A, Rabago D, Zuelsdorff M, Coe C, Miller M, Fleming M. Mindfulness meditation for alcohol relapse prevention: a feasibility pilot study. *J Addict Med.* 2008; 2:165–173.

34. Marlatt GA. Buddhist philosophy and the treatment of addictive behavior. *Cogn Behav Pract.* 2002; 9: 44–49.

35. Teasdale JD. The relationship between cognition and emotion: the mind-in-place in mood disorders. In: Clark DM, Fairburn CG, eds. *Science and Practice of Cognitive Behavior Therapy.* Oxford, England: Oxford University Press; 1997:67–93.

36. Teasdale JD, Segal Z, Williams JMG. How does cognitive therapy prevent depressive relapse and why should attentional control (mindfulness) training help? *Behav Res Ther.* 1995; 33:25–39.

37. Breslin FC, Zack M, McMain S. An information-processing analysis of mindfulness: implications for relapse prevention in the treatment of substance abuse. *Clin Psychol Sci Pract.* 2002; 9:275–299.

38. First MB, Gibbon M, Spitzer RL, Williams JBW. *Structured Clinical Interview for DSM-IV (SCID).* New York: New York State Psychiatric Institute; 1995.

39. Hamilton M. A rating scale for depression. *J Neurol Neurosurg.* 1960; 23: 56–62.

40. Derogatis LR, Melisaratos N. The Brief Symptom Inventory: an introductory report. *Psychol Med.* 1983; 13: 595–605.

41. Sobell LC, Sobell MB. A technique for assessing self-reported alcohol consumption. In: Litten RZ, Allen J, eds. *Measuring Alcohol Consumption: Psychosocial and Biological Methods.* Totowa, NJ: Humana Press; 1992:41–72.

42. Sobell LC, Brown JL, Gloria I, Sobell MB. The reliability of the Alcohol Timeline Followback when administered by telephone and by computer. *Drug Alcohol Depend.* 1996; 42:49–54.

43. Flannery BA, Volpicelli JR, Pettinati HM. Psychometric properties of the Penn Alcohol Craving Scale. *Alcohol Clin Exp Res.* 1999; 23:1289–1295.

44. Blanchard KA, Morgenstern J, Morgan TJ, Labouvie EW, Bux DA. Assessing consequences of substance use: psychometric properties of the inventory of drug use consequences. *Psychol Addict Behav.* 2003; 17:328–331.

45. Miller WR, Tonigan JS, Longabaugh R. *The Drinker Inventory of Consequences (DrInC).* Project MATCH Monograph Series Vol. 4. Mattson ME, ed. Rockville, MD: National Institute on Alcohol Abuse and Alcoholism; 1995.

46. Baer RA, Smith GT, Hopkins J, Krietemeyer J, Toney L. Using self-report assessment methods to explore facets of mindfulness. *Assessment* 2006; 13:27–45.

47. Hayes SC, Strosahl KD, Wilson KG, Bissett RT, Pistorello J, Taormino D, Polusny MA, Dykstra TA, Batten SV, Bergan J, Stewart SH, Zvolensky MJ, Eifert GH, Bond FW, Forsyth JP, Karekla M, McCurry SM. Measuring experiential avoidance: a preliminary test of a working model. *Psychol Rec.* 2004; 54:553–578.

48. Hayes SC, Wilson KG, Gifford EV, Follette VM, Strosahl K. Experiential avoidance and behavioral disorders: a functional dimensional approach to diagnosis and treatment. *J Consult Clin Psychol.* 1996; 64:1152–1168.

49. Kabat-Zinn J. Guided Mindfulness Meditation [audio CD]. Lexington, MA: Sounds True, Incorporated; 2002.

50. Ellis A, MacLaren C. *Rational Emotive Behavior Therapy: A Therapist's Guide.* Atascadero, CA: Impact Publishers; 2005:166.

51. Gorski TT. *The Gorski-Cenaps Model for Recovery and Relapse Prevention.* Independence, MO: Herald House/Independence Press; 2007.

52. Zeger SL, Liang KY. Longitudinal data analysis for discrete and continuous outcomes. *Biometrics* 1986; 42:121–130.

53. StataCorp. Stata Statistical Software: Release 10. College Station, TX: StataCorp; 2007.

54. Neal DJ, Simons JS. Inference in regression models of heavily skewed alcohol use data: a comparison of ordinary least squares, generalized linear models, and bootstrap resampling. *Psychol Addict Behav.* 2007; 21:441–452.

55. Hardin JW, Hilbe JM. *Generalized Estimating Equations.* Boca Raton, FL: Chapman Hall/CRC; 2003.

56. Salim A, MacKinnon A, Christensen H, Griffiths K. Comparison of data analysis strategies for intent-to-treat analysis in pretest-posttest designs with substantial dropout rates. *Psychiatry Res.* 2008; 160: 335–345.

57. Metz K, Stephanie Flöter S, Kröger C, Donath C, Piontek P, Gradl S. Telephone booster sessions for optimizing smoking cessation for patients in rehabilitation centers. *Nicotine Tob Res.* 2007; 9:853–863.

58. Connors GJ, Walitzer KS. Reducing alcohol consumption among heavily drinking women: evaluating the contributions of life-skills training and booster sessions. *J Consult Clin Psychol.* 2001; 3: 447–456.

59. Clark DM, Ball S, Pape D. An experimental investigation of thought suppression. *Behav Res Ther.* 1991; 29: 253–257.

60. Gold DB, Wegner DM. Origins of ruminative thought: trauma, incompleteness, non-disclosure and suppression. *J Appl Soc Psychol.* 1995; 25:1245–1261.

61. Gross JJ, John OP. Individual differences in two emotion regulation processes: implications for affect, relationships, and well-being. *J Pers Soc Psychol.* 2003; 85: 348–362.

62. Wegner DM, Schneider DJ, Carter SR, White TL. Paradoxical effects of thought suppression. *J Pers Soc Psychol.* 1987; 53: 5–13.

63. Wegner DM, Schneider DJ, Knutson B, McMahon SR. Polluting the stream of consciousness: the effects of thought suppression on the mind's environment. *Cognit Ther Res.* 1991; 15: 141–151.

64. Marks I. Behavior therapy for obsessive-compulsive disorder: a decade of progress. *Can J Psychiatry.* 1997; 42:1021–1027.

65. Holzel BK, Ulrich O, Gard T, Hempel HH, Weygandt M, Morgen K. Investigation of mindfulness meditation practitioners with voxel-based morphometry. *Scan* 2008; 3:55–61.

66. Lazar SW, Bush G, Gollup RL, Fricchione GL, Khalsa G, Benson H. Functional brain mapping of the relaxation response and meditation. *Neuroreport* 2000; 11: 1–5.

67. Farrington DP, Petrosino A, Welsh BC. Systematic reviews and cost-benefit analyses of correctional interventions. *Prison J.* 2001; 81:339–359.

Mindfulness Training and Stress Reactivity in Substance Abuse: Results from a Randomized, Controlled Stage I Pilot Study

Judson A. Brewer, MD, PhD

Rajita Sinha, PhD

Justin A. Chen, MD

Ravenna N. Michalsen, MA

Theresa A. Babuscio, MA

Charla Nich, MS

Aleesha Grier, PhD

Keri L. Bergquist, PhD

Deidre L. Reis, PhD

Marc N. Potenza, MD, PhD

Kathleen M. Carroll, PhD

Bruce J. Rounsaville, MD

ABSTRACT. Stress is important in substance use disorders (SUDs). Mindfulness training (MT) has shown promise for stress-related maladies. No studies have compared MT to empirically validated treatments for SUDs. The goals of this study were to assess MT compared to cognitive behavioral

Judson A. Brewer, Rajita Sinha, Justin A. Chen, Ravenna N. Michalsen, Theresa A. Babuscio, Charla Nich, Aleesha Grier, Keri L. Bergquist, Marc N. Potenza, Kathleen M. Carroll, and Bruce J. Rounsaville are affiliated with the Department of Psychiatry, Yale University School of Medicine, New Haven, Connecticut, USA.

Deidre L. Reis is affiliated with the Department of Psychology, Yale University, New Haven, Connecticut, USA.

Rajita Sinha and Marc N. Potenza are also affiliated with the Child Study Center, Yale University School of Medicine, New Haven, Connecticut, USA.

The authors would like to thank the participants and the staff of the Substance Abuse Treatment Unit, without whom this research would not be possible. The authors would like to thank Ginny Morgan, Sarah Bowen, and Jon Kabat-Zinn for helpful discussions regarding adaptations for the MT presented in this paper, and Hedy Kober and Megan McGinn for their help with data input and analysis. The authors would also like to thank the staff of the Yale University Clinical Neuroscience Research Unit, and Psychotherapy Development Center, notably, Zubin Bhagwagar, Robert Malison, Jonas Hannestad, Samuel Ball, and Steve Martino, among others, for helpful discussions. This study was funded by the following grants: NIDA K12-DA00167 (J.A.B.), P50-DA09241 (B.J.R.), R37-DA15969 (K.M.C.), T32-DA007238 (J.A.B.), K05-DA00457 (K.M.C.), K05-DA00089 (B.J.R.), P50-DA16556 (R.S.), K02-DA17232 (R.S.), R01 DA020908 (M.N.P.), RL1 AA017539 (M.N.P.), the U.S. Veterans Affairs New England Mental Illness Research, Education, and Clinical Center (MIRECC) (B.J.R.), and a Varela grant from the Mind and Life Institute (J.A.B.).

Disclosures: The authors have no competing interests.

therapy (CBT) in substance use and treatment acceptability, and specificity of MT compared to CBT in targeting stress reactivity. Thirty-six individuals with alcohol and/or cocaine use disorders were randomly assigned to receive group MT or CBT in an outpatient setting. Drug use was assessed weekly. After treatment, responses to personalized stress provocation were measured. Fourteen individuals completed treatment. There were no differences in treatment satisfaction or drug use between groups. The laboratory paradigm suggested reduced psychological and physiological indices of stress during provocation in MT compared to CBT. This pilot study provides evidence of the feasibility of MT in treating SUDs and suggests that MT may be efficacious in targeting stress.

INTRODUCTION

Considerable evidence has accumulated suggesting that stress exposure can produce an increased arousal state similar to that induced by drug cues (1). Acute stress may increase self-administration of drugs (2,3) and alcohol (4). This is consistent with incentive conditioning models stating that exposure to drug-related cues produces conditioned responses, which in turn can cue subsequent drug-seeking behavior and use (5). Stressful events and psychological distress are frequently cited reasons for relapse to drug use among individuals with substance use disorders (SUDs) (6–8). These data support the hypothesis that mechanisms related to stress are critical in the establishment of addictions and their propagation as chronic disorders (9,10).

Mindfulness-based therapies have shown preliminary evidence for efficacy in the treatment of tobacco, alcohol, and drug use disorders (11–17). For example, Zgierska and colleagues found reductions in anxiety, depression, and stress symptom severity in individuals with alcohol dependence who were enrolled in an 8-week mindfulness meditation intervention after completing an intensive outpatient program (12). Bowen and colleagues also found significant reductions in alcohol and drug use after release from prison in individuals who had undergone a 10-day Vipassana meditation course compared to those who had received treatment as usual (16). However, to date, no randomized trials have compared mindfulness training (MT) to empirically validated treatments for SUDs, such as cognitive behavioral therapy (CBT) (18).

Commonly used behavioral strategies in substance abuse treatment include avoidance of associative cues and suppression of "unwanted" thoughts. However, these strategies may be suboptimal. For example, thought suppression has been shown to lead to *stronger* expectancies after cue exposure (e.g., "alcohol makes me...") (19). Mindfulness-based treatment has been shown to decrease alcohol consumption, which is partially mediated in prisoners by *decreases* in thought suppression indices such as avoidance (13). Also, as mindfulness-based treatments teach an attitude of acceptance/nonjudgment, they may help to mediate the avoidance of negative affective states and thoughts, as has been shown with depression (20–22). Accordingly, MT may be efficacious in treating compulsive drug use—characteristic for addiction—through multiple mechanisms related to stress such as tolerating unpleasant thoughts and emotions.

We describe outcomes from a stage I pilot trial in which we modified an existing manualized version of MT for individuals with SUDs. We evaluated (1) its feasibility by comparing it with empirically validated therapy (CBT), and (2) its specificity toward stress, by evaluating reactivity during stress provocation.

METHODS

Participants

Participants were recruited through media advertisements and clinician referrals of individuals seeking treatment at a community-based

FIGURE 1. Flow of participants through the study protocol. CBT = Cognitive Behavioral Therapy; MT = Mindfulness Training. Laboratory session was performed within two weeks of treatment completion.

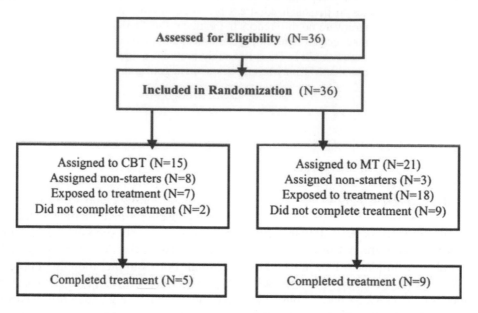

outpatient treatment facility in New Haven, CT. Eligible participants were English-speaking adults who met DSM-IV criteria for alcohol and/or cocaine abuse or dependence in the past year. Individuals were excluded only if they were under 18 years old, currently at clinically significant risk for suicide or homicide, had a current psychotic disorder (assessed by a psychiatrist), had a cognitive impairment precluding completion of study-related activities, or were on beta-blocker treatment.

All of the 36 screened individuals were found eligible and agreed to participate in the study (Figure 1). They provided written informed consent, and were randomly assigned to treatment condition using a 2-choice random number generator (random.org). Of those, 25 were exposed to and 14 completed treatment. Thus, outcome data were available for the 14 treatment completers. Laboratory data were available for 13 treatment completers (collection error rendered data from the 14th person unusable).

Treatments

All participants received weekly group therapy sessions as their sole primary treatment. All treatments were manualized and delivered by PhD-level therapists experienced in CBT or MT, respectively.

CBT was delivered by one therapist over a 12-week period using the National Institute on Drug Abuse CBT manual (23). Sessions were delivered weekly in a continuous fashion such that individuals could enter treatment based on a weekly rolling admission process. Each session lasted roughly 1 hour. Groups were capped at 8 persons to ensure optimal treatment settings.

MT was delivered weekly, over a 9-week period, in a group session format, by one therapist (12 years of mindfulness practice and several years teaching). Groups were also capped at 8 persons to ensure optimal treatment. The MT manual was based on manualized Mindfulness-Based Relapse Prevention (MBRP) program (12,24). Several adaptations to MBRP were made. First, after the first session (renamed Introduction), the 7 sequential sessions were divided into 2 4-week modules that could be completed in either order (Introduction, then Module 1, then Module 2 or Introduction, then Module 2, then Module 1). This was done to assess "real-world" delivery of the treatment by providing minimal waiting time for individuals to enter treatment. Module 1 included MBRP sessions 2, 6, and 7, and, in addition, a session that specifically targeted working with anger as a trigger for stress, drug use, or relapse (25), and instruction for using loving-kindness techniques to facilitate working with difficult emotions (26). Module 2 included MBRP sessions 3, 4, 5, and 8. Second, the yoga meditation was removed to decrease confounding, yoga-specific effects; yoga may have beneficial effects as a stand-alone treatment on stress reduction and drug use (27,28). Third, weekly sessions were shortened to approximately 1 hour (mainly by shortening the guided meditation exercises). This was done to assess whether shorter sessions would be sufficient for individuals to attain adequate mindfulness skills for benefits to be seen, and to mimic as closely as possible, group CBT sessions.

Assessments

The *Structural Clinical Interview for DSM-IV* (SCID) alcohol and drug modules were administered at baseline only to establish SUD-related diagnoses (29). Diagnoses were confirmed by a psychiatrist. All other measures were collected at least at baseline, weekly (as noted below) and upon treatment completion, which was roughly 9 weeks after treatment initiation for the MT and 12 weeks after treatment initiation for the CBT group.

The *Substance Use Calendar* was administered at baseline (past month) and weekly during treatment and measured in standardized drinks/day for alcohol (1 oz) and grams/day for cocaine (30). Participant self-reports of drug use were verified by random breathalyzer for alcohol and urine toxicology screens for drug use (approximately every 2 weeks). One hundred percent of the breathalyzer and 98.4% (62/63) of the urine specimens were consistent with self-reports.

The *Five Facet Mindfulness Questionnaire* (FFMQ) was administered at baseline and treatment completion to assess mindfulness skills acquisition (increased scores denote more skill acquisition) (31,32).

The *Treatment Credibility Score* (TCS) questionnaire was administered at treatment completion. It consisted of questions evaluating, using a 5-point Likert scale, how agreeable and practical treatment was both for drug use and symptoms of depression and anxiety.

The *Differential Emotion Scale* (DES) was used during the laboratory session to assess patterns of emotions after stress provocation (33).

Laboratory Paradigm

Within 2 weeks of treatment completion, subjects participated in an 1-hour laboratory session that included 2 imagery conditions: a neutral-relaxing and stress as previously described (34–37). In a separate session several weeks prior to the laboratory session, imagery scripts were developed for each subject for the stress and neutral-relaxing situations as previously described (34–37). Each script was edited by 2 researchers with multiple years of experience recording and editing imagery scripts (K.L.B. and R.S.) to ensure that personalized scripts were standardized in length and content type. These researchers were blinded to treatment group.

Physiological measurements were recorded using a Biopac MP100 system running AcqKnowledge 3.9 software (Biopac Systems, USA), the Biopac electrodermal activity amplifier module (Galvanic Skin Response [GSR] 100c) set at a channel sampling rate of 31 Hz and a gain of 5 μSiemens (μS) per volt (resulting in a resolution of 0.0015 μS), and the electrocardiogram (ECG) amplifier (ECG 100c) set at a channel sampling rate of 1000 Hz for the laboratory session.

The order of the stress and neutral-relaxing imagery scripts was randomized.

Subjective responses after each script were recorded on a laptop computer using ePrime software (Psychology Software Tools, USA). After each imagery script, participants rated how "clearly and vividly" they were able to imagine the scenario on a 10-point Likert scale. Average vividness ratings were 8.1 $\pm$ 1.1 and 8.6 $\pm$ 0.5 for stress imagery, and average vividness ratings were 8.0 $\pm$ 1.1 and 8.2 $\pm$ 0.4 for neutral imagery for MT and CBT groups, respectively. Participants then rated their anxiety and drug/alcohol cravings on a 10-point Likert scale, and completed the DES questionnaire for each imagery condition.

Data Analysis

Analysis of variance (ANOVA) was performed per protocol for between-group comparisons of drug use and scores on the FFMQ and TCS (SPSS 16). Chi-square analysis was used for treatment retention. DES, anxiety, and drug craving Likert scores were compared by 2-tailed t tests. ANOVA was used to evaluate GSR differences by treatment condition (between subjects) and testing condition (within subjects). Within-subject ANOVAs evaluated influences of sympathetic and vagal tone, with treatment condition, testing condition, and the interaction of treatment and testing condition as the predictors using heart rate variability (HRV) power algorithms (38). For the most part, the self-report outcomes did not violate the assumption of normality (11 of 12 items: Shapiro-Wilks >.05). Although a few of the physiological variables were non-normally distributed (maximum stress heart rate [HR], neutral sympathetic/vagal ratio), the complexity of the analysis was not one that could be handled with nonparametric tests. Thus, ANOVA was used as noted above.

Data are reported as mean ± standard deviation. Effect sizes are reported as partial η^2. Level of significance was defined as P value less than .05.

RESULTS

Group Description

As shown in Table 1, most of the randomized participants were male (72%), single or divorced (76%), did not have a college degree (76%), and were not employed full-time (72%). The majority met the DSM-IV criteria for alcohol dependence (68%) and/or cocaine dependence (48%). Analysis of variance and chi-square analysis indicated no significant differences by treatment condition except marital status (57% married in CBT versus 6% married in MT, $P = .02$). No differences in baseline drug or alcohol use were found between treatment completers ($N = 14$) and noncompleters ($N = 22$). Among treatment completers, although substance use in the

month prior to treatment initiation was reported by twice as many subjects in the MT (8/9) compared to the CBT group (2/5), it did not differ by group status at baseline (Table 1).

Feasibility: Treatment Retention and Satisfaction

To evaluate the feasibility and acceptability of MT relative to CBT, we compared treatment retention (defined as treatment drop-out) and satisfaction across the two treatment conditions. Of the 36 individuals who entered the study, 9/21 (43%) completed MT, whereas 5/15 (33%) completed CBT ($P = .56$; Figure 1). Participants who initiated treatment ($N = 25$) attended 65% of sessions in MT versus 34% of sessions in CBT group ($F = 4.89$, $P = .04$). Participants who completed treatment ($N = 14$) in both groups rated their treatments as highly satisfactory as assessed by TCS (4.2 ± 0.5 versus 4.4 ± .5 of 5, $P = .37$).

Substance Use Outcomes

No differences in alcohol and cocaine use were found during the treatment period but trended toward favoring the CBT group (in MT versus CBT groups, self-reported % days of cocaine use: 5.4 ± 8 versus 0.0 ± 0.0, $P = .17$; and alcohol use: 24.3 ± 28 versus 0.0 ± 0.0, $P = .09$). No side effects or adverse events were noted.

Specificity of MT: Effects of Treatment on Mindfulness Skills Acquisition and Implementation

To determine whether our paradigm adequately fostered mindfulness skills development, we measured the FFMQ scores before and after treatment. At baseline, there were no observed differences in the FFMQ between groups regarding all enrolled participants (MT = 127 ± 26, CBT = 123 ± 23, $P = .64$) as well as treatment completers only (MT = 122 ± 26, CBT = 119 ± 29, $P = .82$).

Treatment completers in both MT and CBT groups showed significantly increased FFMQ scores over time. Although participants in the MT group showed tendency toward greater

TABLE 1. Baseline Demographics and Substance Use

	CBT ($N = 7$)		MT ($N = 18$)		Total ($N = 25$)		P
Sex	N (%)		N (%)		N (%)		
Male	5 (71.4)		13 (72.2)		18 (72)		.968
Female	2 (28.6)		5 (27.8)		7 (28)		
Race							
White	6 (85.7)		10 (55.6)		16 (64)		.213
Black	0		6 (33.3)		6 (24)		
Hispanic	1 (14.3)		2 (11.1)		3 (12)		
Education level							
College or more	4 (57.1)		9 (50)		13 (52)		.748
High school/GED or Partial HS	3 (42.9)		9 (50)		12 (48)		
Marital status							
Never married	2 (28.6)		11 (61.1)		13 (52)		.015
Married	4 (57.1)		1 (5.6)		5 (20)		
Divorced/separated	1 (14.3)		6 (33.3)		7 (28)		
Employment Status							
Employed	4 (57.1)		11 (61.1)		15 (60)		.856
Unemployed	3 (42.9)		7 (38.9)		10 (40)		
Alcohol DSM IV Diagnosis							
Dependence	6 (85.7)		13 (72.2)		19 (76)		.478
Cocaine DSM IV Diagnosis							
Dependence	2 (28.6)		10 (55.6)		12 (48)		.225
MJ positive baseline	0		3 (21.4)		3 (15)		.219
Cocaine positive baseline	0		3 (21.4)		3 (15)		.219
	Mean + SD	N	Mean + SD	N	Mean + SD	N	P
Age (years)	45 + 13.5	7	35.6 + 10.4	18	38.2 + 11.9	25	.075
Years of Education	13.7 + 2.2	7	13.1 + 2.4	18	13.2 + 2.3	25	.541
Days of alcohol use in the past 28 days	0	5	.06 + .24	17	.05 + .21	22	.600
Days of marijuana use in the past 28 days	0	5	.19 + .40	16	.14 + .36	21	.320
Days of cocaine use in the past 28 days	0	5	.06 + .24	17	.05 + .21	22	.600
Days of tobacco use in the past 28 days	.20 + .44	5	.5S + .52	15	.45 + .51	20	.215
Number of lifetime drug treatments	1.6 + 2.5	7	2.2 + 1.9	18	2 + 2.1	25	.492

Note. GED = general educational development diploma; HS = high school; DSM = *Diagnostic and Statistical Manual of Mental Disorders*; MJ = marijuana.

overall increases in FFMQ scores compared to CBT after treatment, these differences did not reach statistical significance (MT $= 144 \pm 18$; CBT $= 131 \pm 27$, $P = .04$ by time, $P = .54$ group by time).

Specificity of MT: Subjective and Objective Responses to Stress Provocation

To determine if MT differentially influenced psychological responses to stress, we compared responses to a personalized stress challenge in treatment completers. Participants who received MT reported significantly attenuated anxiety in both anxiety Likert scales and DES anxious subscale scores (Stress minus Neutral Anxiety: 1.5 ± 2.1 versus 4.6 ± 1.5, $P = .01$, Figure 2a; DES: 1.5 ± 3.9 versus 7.0 ± 3.8, $P = .03$, Figure 3). Though not statistically significant, individuals receiving MT also reported about half the stress-induced drug craving compared to those receiving CBT (1.1 ± 3.7 versus 2.0 ± 3.1, $P = .65$, Figure 2b). These attenuations were echoed in several other negative emotion scores, such as sadness, anger, and fear (Figure 3).

We also sought to determine if MT, compared to CBT, differentially influenced physiological measures of stress. As expected, we found large differences in galvanic skin responses between stress and neutral stories; however, they were not different between groups (MT $= 10.0 \pm 8.2$ versus 4.5 ± 7.4; CBT $= 7.0 \pm 6.4$ versus 0.8 ± 1.1, $F = 12.36$, $P = .01$ for condition). However, no increases in maximum HR were seen in the MT

FIGURE 2. Anxiety and drug craving during stress provocation (MT, $n = 8$; CBT, $n = 5$). Y-axis denotes reported anxiety scores after listening to personalized neutral or stressful stories. (a) Anxiety severity scores: far right indicates normalized scores (stress minus neutral). (b) Normalized drug craving severity scores (stress minus neutral). $**P = .01$ for the difference between treatment groups.

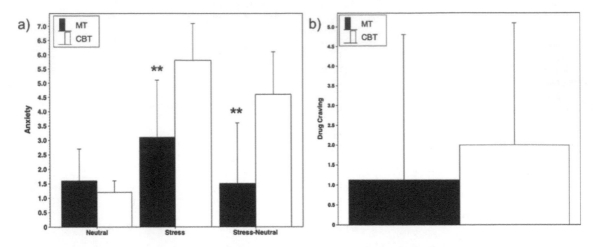

FIGURE 3. Emotional responses during stress provocation (MT, $n = 8$; CBT, $n = 5$). Y-axis denotes normalized Differential Emotion Scale scores after stress provocation (stress minus neutral). $*P \leq .05$ between treatment groups.

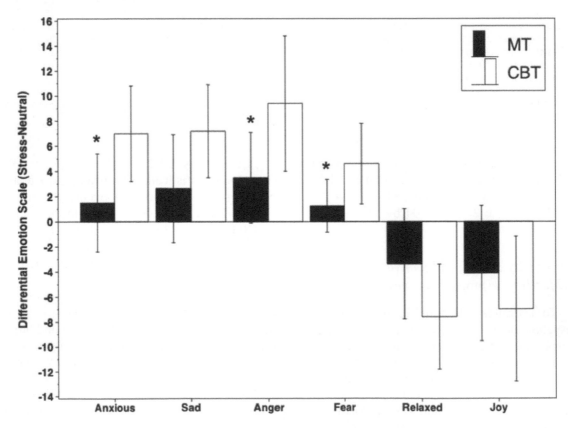

FIGURE 4. Maximum heart rate and autonomic nervous system tone during stress provocation (MT, $n = 8$; CBT, $n = 5$). (a) Maximum heart rate during neutral and stressful stories. (b) Percent change in sympathetic/vagal ratio during stress versus neutral stories. *$F = 7.97$ and $P = .02$ by treatment condition.

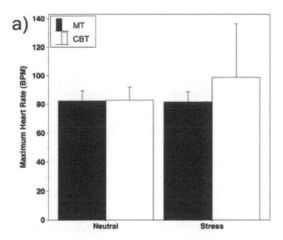

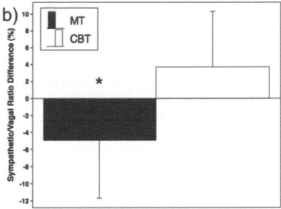

group during stress, where these expected increases were observed in the CBT group (MT = 81.4 ± 7.0 versus CBT = 98.7 ± 37.6, $P = 0.19$, Figure 4a). Although these findings were not significant, the partial η^2 indicated this effect size to be large (.15). Corresponding differences were seen in heart rate variability measures: individuals in the MT group showed decreased sympathetic/vagal ratios compared to the CBT group (MT = $4.0 \pm .5$ versus CBT = $4.2 \pm .2$, $F = 7.97$, $P = .02$, effect size = .42, Figure 4b).

DISCUSSION

This pilot trial sought to evaluate the feasibility and specificity of 9-week-long MT versus 12-week-long CBT group therapies for individuals with alcohol and/or cocaine dependence. During the treatment period, MT did not significantly differ from CBT in participant retention, treatment satisfaction, or frequency of substance use. However, those who completed MT demonstrated attenuated psychological and physiological responses to stress provocation compared to CBT group. This is, to our knowledge, the first randomized clinical trial comparing MT to an empirically validated treatment for SUDs, such as CBT, and the first to assess

responses to stress provocation in laboratory settings in this clinical population.

Treatment Implications

There are several important, clinically relevant implications of this pilot trial. First, the presented data suggest that MT may be a viable, possibly comparable treatment option to CBT regarding treatment feasibility, acceptability, and even outcomes. Of note, MT has not previously been compared head-to-head to CBT in treatment-seeking individuals with SUDs.

Mindfulness training can be conceptualized to target one's relationship with thoughts (i.e., the *process* of events arising), whereas a primary focus of CBT is to change the *content* of thoughts (please see (39) for a full discussion). From this, one might ask if an ability to notice one's thought patterns (i.e., mindfulness) is a prerequisite to changing them, and consequently, whether these techniques might be combined for greater efficacy. Indeed, work with depressed individuals has shown robust effects of treatments that teach mindfulness while incorporating cognitive techniques (Mindfulness-Based Cognitive Therapy) (20,21).

A previous pilot study of individuals from the general population recruited for a "stress-reduction" (Mindfulness-Based Stress Reduction [MBSR]) versus a "stress-management"

(CBT-based stress reduction) class found between-group differences in self-reported health measures such as pain, and energy, but similar effects on perceived stress, depression, and well-being (40). They also found an expected increase in self-reported mindfulness in the MBSR group, but a decrease in this measure in the CBT-based stress reduction group. They suggested that this difference may be due to participants' efforts to "change and control thought and feelings may reduce the awareness of cues ..." (40). We did not find decreases in self-reported mindfulness in our CBT population, but instead found trends toward increased mindfulness. Though direct comparisons cannot be drawn between these studies due to differences in target populations and treatments, future studies will help to differentiate the effects of CBT on self-reported mindfulness acquisition.

Second, the length of each MT treatment session was significantly shortened compared to standard mindfulness-based programs, and MT was delivered in a modular rather than sequential format. These changes were meant to facilitate subject retention/treatment compliance, and to allow for a more timely and "flexible" subject study entry.

"Standard" mindfulness training programs, such as MBSR, usually utilize 8 sequential sessions of approximately 2-hour duration each, delivered once a week for 8 weeks. Such "standard" training has been shown to result in increased self-reported degree of mindfulness (successful "acquisition"), which, in turn, has recently been documented to correlate with psychological functioning and medical symptom reduction (41). The "dose-response" curve for mindfulness acquisition and MT treatment delivered in a block design—as implemented in the current study—has not been previously evaluated. Our data suggest that shorter-than-standard MT sessions may still provide sufficient training to establish efficacy. They also suggest that a modular format is a viable MT delivery option. Developing treatments that are shorter than typical mindfulness-based approaches may also be more cost-efficient for community clinics and less of a time "burden" for patients. Additionally, modular formats may decrease the number of trained therapists needed to deliver a given

intervention as has been shown with dialectical behavioral therapy programs (42).

Stress and Addiction

Our stress paradigm provided robust psychological and physiological responses, as evidenced by increases in emotional and craving ratings and GSR and HR measures. Importantly, the number of GSRs increased in stress stories in both groups, which suggests that all individuals engaged in these stories, and thus, did not employ avoidance or suppression strategies, which have been shown to lead to increased numbers of intrusive drug-related thoughts (43) and have been linked to worse outcomes in SUDs (44,45). Importantly, we found that, compared to CBT group, subjective measures of stress were reduced in MT during stress provocation. This is consistent with the conceptual framework behind mindfulness techniques suggesting that MT fosters an engaged but *nonattached* participation in events (46).

Previously, we and others have found increases in HR indices in individuals with SUDs undergoing stress (1,47,48). In this study, we found an attenuation of HR increases with MT, which provides objective corroboration of individuals' report of attenuated anxiety and negative emotions. These findings are important for individuals with SUDs as self-report measures can be problematic with regard to accuracy due to psychological defense mechanisms (such as denial) coming into play.

The autonomic nervous system (ANS) is important for psychological and physiological allostasis (49–52). In healthy individuals, the heart is under tonic, parasympathetic inhibitory control. This allows for adaptive responses to environmental conditions given the short timecourse of parasympathic effects (milliseconds) compared to sympathetic effects (seconds) (53). ANS imbalance, often characterized by predominance of the sympathetic ANS, has been linked to a range of pathological conditions (54). In this study, we found a decreased sympathetic/vagal ratio in participants in the MT compared to the CBT group. This finding is consistent with the idea that MT promotes a decentered stance toward environmental stimuli: as individuals are able to engage but are not "caught up" in thoughts or emotions, they are more able to adapt to changing internal and external environmental cues and conditions. As vagal tone has been shown to be a peripheral indicator of prefrontal cortical control of downstream sympathetic responses (e.g., anxiety and/or fear) (55), decreases in the sympathetic/vagal ratio also suggest the possibility of prefrontal cortical circuits playing a mechanistic role in MT's mediation of stress. This is an intriguing possibility as prefrontal cortical activation during a cognitive control task (Stroop) has been shown to be associated with improved treatment outcomes in cocaine-dependent individuals (56). Future studies using functional magnetic resonance imaging may help determine specific brain regions that may be altered by MT and how this may affect individual responses to stress.

Strengths and Limitations

Strengths of this trial include the random assignment of a diverse group of participants from a community clinic, the presence of an active comparison group, and the use of both self-reported and objective, validated outcome measures, including a robust laboratory stress paradigm that utilized discrete psychological and physiological measures.

This study has several limitations as well. In particular, the sample size was small and outcome data were collected from the minority of individuals in both conditions (those who completed treatment). The assessment period was limited to pre-, during-, and post-intervention only; it is possible that longer follow-up periods could have yielded different results. Also, it included a heterogeneous population both in regard to SUDs (alcohol and/or cocaine) and drug use status at study entry, though this arguably provided greater ecological validity. This, in the context of a large dropout rate, may have also confounded interpretation of substance use outcomes, as individuals that may have done poorly with treatment, may have also differentially dropped out, leaving a "homogeneous" population of treatment-satisfied abstainers for comparisons. Further, though not statistically different, one may speculate that the higher amount of drug use prior to treatment may suggest a "sicker" cohort at treatment onset in the MT group. Additionally, this study was performed at a single site using single therapists for each condition, and measures of treatment fidelity or discriminability were not conducted. Thus, the amount/quality of treatment was not objectively assessed. Finally, the treatments were of unequal length (9 MT versus 12 CBT weekly sessions), and thus results may have been confounded by natural progression of disease or "dose" of treatment.

In conclusions, results of this pilot study suggest that MT may have promise as a component of addiction treatment and further studies evaluating MT effects on stress reactivity and other substance use related outcomes are warranted.

REFERENCES

1. Sinha R, Talih M, Malison R, Cooney N, Anderson GM, Kreek MJ. Hypothalamic-pituitary-adrenal axis and sympatho-adreno-medullary responses during stress-induced and drug cue-induced cocaine craving states. *Psychopharmacology (Berl).* 2003;170:62–72.

2. Cabib S, Puglisi-Allegra S, Genua C, Simon H, Le Moal M, Piazza PV. Dose-dependent aversive and rewarding effects of amphetamine as revealed by a new place conditioning apparatus. *Psychopharmacology (Berl).* 1996;125:92–96.

3. Kalivas PW, Duffy P. Similar effects of daily cocaine and stress on mesocorticolimbic dopamine neurotransmission in the rat. *Biol Psychiatry.* 1989;25:913–928.

4. Volpicelli JR. Uncontrollable events and alcohol drinking. *Br J Addict.* 1987;82:381–392.

5. O'Brien CP, Childress AR, Ehrman R, Robbins SJ. Conditioning factors in drug abuse: can they explain compulsion? *J Psychopharmacol.* 1998;12:15–22.

6. Marlatt GA, Gordon JR. *Relapse Prevention: Maintenance Strategies in the Treatment of Addictive Behaviors.* New York: Guilford Press; 1985.

7. Brownell KD, Marlatt GA, Lichtenstein E, Wilson GT. Understanding and preventing relapse. *Am Psychol.* 1986;41:765–782.

8. Wallace BC. Psychological and environmental determinants of relapse in crack cocaine smokers. *J Subst Abuse Treat.* 1989;6:95–106.

9. Sinha R, Fox HC, Hong KA, Bergquist K, Bhagwagar Z, Siedlarz KM. Enhanced negative emotion and alcohol craving, and altered physiological responses following stress and cue exposure in alcohol dependent individuals. *Neuropsychopharmacology.* 2008;34:1198–1208.

10. Brady KT, Sinha R. Co-occurring mental and substance use disorders: the neurobiological effects of chronic stress. *Am J Psychiatry.* 2005;162:1483–1493.

11. Hoppes K. The application of mindfulness-based cognitive interventions in the treatment of co-occurring addictive and mood disorders. *CNS Spectr.* 2006;11:829–851.

12. Zgierska A, Rabago D, Zuelsdorff M, Coe C, Miller M, Fleming M. Mindfulness meditation for alcohol relapse prevention: a feasibility pilot study. *J Addict Med.* 2008;2:165–73.

13. Bowen S, Witkiewitz K, Dillworth TM, Marlatt GA. The role of thought suppression in the relationship between mindfulness meditation and alcohol use. *Addict Behav.* 2007;32:2324–2328.

14. Davis JM, Fleming MF, Bonus KA, Baker TB. A pilot study on mindfulness based stress reduction for smokers. *BMC Comple Altern Med.* 2007;7:2.

15. Marlatt GA. Buddhist philosophy and the treatment of addictive behavior. *Cogn Behav Pract.* 2002;9:44–50.

16. Bowen S, Witkiewitz K, Dillworth TM, Chawla N, Simpson TL, Ostafin BD, Larimer ME, Blume AW, Parks GA, Marlatt GA. Mindfulness meditation and substance use in an incarcerated population. *Psychol Addict Behav.* 2006;20:343–7.

17. Marlatt G, Witkiewitz K, Dillworth TM, Bowen SW, Parks GA, Macpherson LM, Lonczak HS, Larimer ME, Simpson T, Blume AW, Crutcher R. Vipassana meditation as a treatment for alcohol and drug use disorders. In: Hayes S, Follette VM, Linehan MM, eds. *Mindfulness and Acceptance.* New York: Guilford Press; 2004:261–287.

18. Dutra L, Stathopoulou G, Basden SL, Leyro TM, Powers MB, Otto MW. A meta-analytic review of psychosocial interventions for substance use disorders. *Am J Psychiatry.* 2008;165:179–187.

19. Palfai TP, Monti PM, Colby SM, Rohsenow DJ. Effects of suppressing the urge to drink on the accessibility of alcohol outcome expectancies. *Behav Res Ther.* 1997;35:59–65.

20. Ma SH, Teasdale JD. Mindfulness-based cognitive therapy for depression: replication and exploration of differential relapse prevention effects. *J Consult Clin Psychol.* 2004;72:31–40.

21. Teasdale JD, Segal ZV, Williams JM, Ridgeway VA, Soulsby JM, Lau MA. Prevention of relapse/recurrence in major depression by mindfulness-based cognitive therapy. *J Consult Clin Psychol.* 2000;68:615–623.

22. Teasdale JD, Moore RG, Hayhurst H, Pope M, Williams S, Segal ZV. Metacognitive awareness and prevention of relapse in depression: empirical evidence. *J Consult Clin Psychol.* 2002;70:275–287.

23. Carroll KM. A cognitive-behavioral approach: treating cocaine addiction. In: *Therapy Manuals for Drug Abuse.* Vol. 98–4308. Rockville, MD: National Institute on Druge Abuse; 1998.

24. Witkiewitz K, Marlatt GA, Walker D. Mindfulness-based relapse prevention for alcohol and substance use disorders. *J Cogn Psychother.* 2005;19:211–228.

25. Roth B. Incorporating an experiential exploration of anger and forgiveness into the MBSR curriculum. Presented at the Center for Mindfulness Annual Scientific Conference, 2006, Worchester, MA.

26. Gunaratana H. *Mindfulness in Plain English.* Somerville, MA: Wisdom Publications; 2002.

27. Kirkwood G, Rampes H, Tuffrey V, Richardson J, Pilkington K. Yoga for anxiety: a systematic review of the research evidence. *Br J Sports Med.* 2005;39:884–891, discussion 891.

28. Shaffer HJ, LaSalvia TA, Stein JP. Comparing Hatha yoga with dynamic group psychotherapy for enhancing methadone maintenance treatment: a randomized clinical trial. *Altern Ther Health Med.* 1997;3:57–66.

29. Spitzer RL, Williams JB, Gibbon M, First MB. The structured clinical interview for DSM-III-R (SCID). I: History, rationale, and description. *Arch Gen Psychiatry.* 1992;49:624–629.

30. Miller WR, Del Boca FK. Measurement of drinking behavior using the Form 90 family of instruments. *J Stud Alcohol.* [*Special Issue: Alcoholism Treatment Matching Research: Methodological and Clinical Approaches.*] 1994;(Suppl 12):112–118.

31. Baer RA, Smith GT, Hopkins J. Krietemeyer J, Toney L, Using self-report assessment methods to explore facets of mindfulness. *Assessment.* 2006;13:27–45.

32. Baer RA, Smith GT, Lykins E, Button D, Krietemeyer J, Sauer S, Walsh E, Duggan D, Williams JMG. Construct validity of the five facet mindfulness questionnaire in meditating and nonmeditating samples. *Assessment.* 2008;15(3):329–342. 1073191107313003.

33. Izard C. *Patterns of Emotions: A New Analysis of Anxiety and Depression.* New York: Academic Press; 1972.

34. Sinha R, Lacadie C, Skudlarski P, Fulbright RK, Rounsaville BJ, Kosten TR, Wexler BE. Neural activity associated with stress-induced cocaine craving: a functional magnetic resonance imaging study. *Psychopharmacology (Berl).* 2005;183:171–180.

35. Sinha R, Garcia M, Paliwal P, Kreek MJ, Rounsaville BJ. Stress-induced cocaine craving and hypothalamic-pituitary-adrenal responses are predictive of cocaine relapse outcomes. *Arch Gen Psychiatry.* 2006;63:324–331.

36. Sinha R, Fuse T, Aubin LR, O'Malley SS. Psychological stress, drug-related cues and cocaine craving. *Psychopharmacology (Berl).* 2000;152:140–148.

37. Sinha R, Catapano D, O'Malley S. Stress-induced craving and stress response in cocaine dependent individuals. *Psychopharmacology (Berl).* 1999;142:343–351.

38. Kleiger RE, Stein PK, Bigger JT Jr. Heart rate variability: measurement and clinical utility. *Ann Noninvasive Electrocardiol.* 2005;10:88–101.

39. Gilpin R. The use of Theravada Buddhist practices and perspectives in mindfulness-based cognitive therapy. *Contemporary Buddhism.* 2008;9:223–251.

40. Smith BW, Shelley BM, Dalen J, Wiggins K, Tooley E, Bernard J. A pilot study comparing the effects of

mindfulness-based and cognitive-behavioral stress reduction. *J Altern Comple Med.* 2008;14:251–258.

41. Carmody J, Baer RA. Relationships between mindfulness practice and levels of mindfulness, medical and psychological symptoms and well-being in a mindfulness-based stress reduction program. *J Behav Med.* 2008;31:23–33.

42. Linehan MM, Schmidt H, 3rd, Dimeff LA, Craft JC, Kanter J, Comtois KA. Dialectical behavior therapy for patients with borderline personality disorder and drug-dependence. *Am J Addict.* 1999;8:279–292.

43. Salkovskis PM, Reynolds M. Thought suppression and smoking cessation. *Behav Res Ther.* 1994;32:193–201.

44. Leary MR, Adams CE, Tate EB. Hypo-egoic self-regulation: exercising self-control by diminishing the influence of the self. *J Personality.* 2006;74:1803–1832.

45. Wilson KG, Murrell AR. Values work in acceptance and commitment therapy: setting a course for behavioral treatment. In: Hayes S, Follette VM, Linehan MM, eds. *Mindfulness and Acceptance.* New York: Guilford Press; 2004:120–151.

46. Shapiro SL, Bootzin RR, Figueredo AJ, Lopez AM, Schwartz GE. The efficacy of mindfulness-based stress reduction in the treatment of sleep disturbance in women with breast cancer: an exploratory study. *J Psychosomatic Res.* 2003;54:85–91.

47. Back SE, Brady KT, Jackson JL, Salstrom S, Zinzow H. Gender differences in stress reactivity among cocaine-dependent individuals. *Psychopharmacology (Berl).* 2005;180:169–76.

48. Back SE, Waldrop AE, Saladin ME, Yeatts SD, Simpson A, McRae AL, Upadhyaya HP, Contini Sisson R, Spratt EG, Allen J, Kreek MJ, Brady KT. Effects of gender and cigarette smoking on reactivity to psychological and pharmacological stress provocation. *Psychoneuroendocrinology.* 2008;33:560–568.

49. Goldstein DS, McEwen B. Allostasis, homeostats, and the nature of stress. *Stress.* 2002;5:55–58.

50. McEwen BS. Stress, adaptation, and disease. Allostasis and allostatic load. *Ann N Y Acad Sci.* 1998;840:33–44.

51. McEwen BS. Protection and damage from acute and chronic stress: allostasis and allostatic overload and relevance to the pathophysiology of psychiatric disorders. *Ann N Y Acad Sci.* 2004;1032:1–7.

52. McEwen BS, Wingfield JC. The concept of allostasis in biology and biomedicine. *Horm Behav.* 2003;43:2–15.

53. Thayer JF, Brosschot JF. Psychosomatics and psychopathology: looking up and down from the brain. *Psychoneuroendocrinology.* 2005;30:1050–1058.

54. Thayer JF, Sternberg E. Beyond heart rate variability: vagal regulation of allostatic systems. *Ann N Y Acad Sci.* 2006;1088:361–372.

55. Amat J, Baratta MV, Paul E, Bland ST, Watkins LR, Maier SF. Medial prefrontal cortex determines how stressor controllability affects behavior and dorsal raphe nucleus. *Nat Neurosci.* 2005;8:365–371.

56. Brewer JA, Worhunsky PD, Carroll KM, Rounsaville BJ, Potenza MN. Pretreatment brain activation during stroop task is associated with outcomes in cocaine-dependent patients. *Biol Psychiatry.* 2008;64:998–1004.

Associations of Mindfulness with Nicotine Dependence, Withdrawal, and Agency

Jennifer Irvin Vidrine, PhD
Michael S. Businelle, PhD
Paul Cinciripini, PhD
Yisheng Li, PhD
Marianne T. Marcus, EdD, RN
Andrew J. Waters, PhD
Lorraine R. Reitzel, PhD
David W. Wetter, PhD

ABSTRACT. Quitting smoking is a major life stressor that results in numerous aversive consequences, including persistently increased level of post-cessation negative affect and relapse. The identification of factors that may enhance behavioral and emotional regulation after quitting may be useful in enhancing quit rates and preventing relapse. One factor broadly linked with behavioral and emotional regulation is mindfulness. This study examined baseline associations of mindfulness with demographic variables, smoking history, dependence, withdrawal severity, and agency among 158 smokers enrolled in a cessation trial. Results indicated that mindfulness was negatively associated with level of nicotine dependence and withdrawal severity, and positively associated with a sense of agency regarding cessation. Moreover, mindfulness remained significantly associated with these measures even after controlling for key demographic variables. Results suggest that low level of mindfulness may be an important predictor of vulnerability to relapse among adult smokers preparing to quit; thus, mindfulness-based interventions may enhance cessation.

Jennifer Irvin Vidrine, Michael S. Businelle, Lorraine R. Reitzel, and David W. Wetter are affiliated with the Department of Health Disparities Research, The University of Texas M. D. Anderson Cancer Center, Houston, Texas, USA.

Paul Cinciripini is affiliated with the Department of Behavioral Science, The University of Texas M. D. Anderson Cancer Center, Houston, Texas, USA.

Yisheng Li is affiliated with the Department of Biostatistics, The University of Texas M. D. Anderson Cancer Center, Houston, Texas, USA.

Marianne T. Marcus is affiliated with the Center for Substance Abuse Prevention, Education and Research, School of Nursing, University of Texas Health Science Center, Houston, Texas, USA.

Andrew J. Waters is affiliated with the Department of Medical and Clinical Psychology, Uniformed Services University of the Health Sciences, Bethesda, Maryland, USA.

This research and preparation of this article were supported by grants from the National Institute on Drug Abuse (R01DA018875, PI: D.W.W.), the Centers for Disease Control and Prevention (K01CD000086, PI: J.I.V.; K01DP001120, PI: L.R.R.) and the National Cancer Institute (R25CA57730).

INTRODUCTION

Tobacco use is the leading cause of preventable morbidity and mortality in the United States (1). Unfortunately, long-term quit rates are low. This is not surprising given that quitting smoking is a major life stressor, resulting in numerous aversive consequences such as mood and sleep disturbance, and cognitive and psychomotor deficits (2). These consequences can be generally characterized as behavioral or emotional. One factor broadly and consistently linked with behavioral and emotion regulation is degree of mindfulness (3). Mindfulness reflects an intentional awareness of internal and external stimuli occurring in the present moment. A key characteristic of mindfulness is that by simply noticing emotions, cognitions, perceptions, and sensations, as they are happening, in a nonjudgmental manner, individuals learn over time that these phenomena are transient and that they are not compelled to impulsively react (4).

Although the evidence is limited, several pilot studies have provided preliminary support for the efficacy of mindfulness-based treatments for smoking cessation (5–7). In addition, degree of mindfulness was found to be negatively associated with the frequency of heavy drinking (8). The focus of the current study is on potential associations of degree of trait mindfulness with nicotine dependence, withdrawal severity, and a sense of agency regarding cessation. These outcomes are of interest because they were found to be predictive of smoking cessation and relapse.

Nicotine dependence has been established as the primary factor responsible for the maintenance of smoking, and dependence severity strongly predicts withdrawal severity and relapse (9). Recent conceptualizations have emphasized the multidimensional nature of dependence, which encompasses factors such as negative (e.g., smoking to alleviate negative affect) and positive (e.g., smoking to enhance mood) reinforcement, and automaticity (e.g., automatically reaching for a cigarette after quitting and disposing of cigarettes). Degree of mindfulness and level of nicotine dependence are hypothesized to be related because mindfulness reduces both self-report and objective indices of negative affect and stress (10), and is associated with enhanced positive affect (11). That is, greater mindfulness is hypothesized to attenuate levels of dependence via its influence on reducing negative affect. Given that affect-related constructs are consistently and very powerfully related to relapse (12), mindfulness may impact cessation outcomes through its effects on enhancing emotional regulation. This hypothesis is modeled after Baker and colleagues' reformulation of the negative reinforcement model of drug addiction, which proposes that negative affect is the most important motivational factor driving continued addictive drug use (13).

Mindfulness is also hypothesized to impact dependence through its effects on enhancing attentional control and reducing automaticity. This is consistent with theory and empirical data indicating that mindfulness increases the ability to disengage attention from problematic stimuli (14). Tiffany's cognitive processing model of drug craving posits that drug use behavior becomes largely automatized over time and relapse occurs when individuals are not able to effectively impede automatized smoking routines (15). Smokers governed largely by automaticity may have greater difficulty interrupting smoking patterns and, thus, be more dependent. This has direct implications for cessation because greater automaticity of smoking predicts relapse (16). Thus, more mindful smokers may be able to respond to difficult situations in more flexible and adaptive ("mindful") ways rather than by relying on automatic responses that are more likely to lead to relapse.

Nicotine withdrawal severity is an important outcome because it is a critical hallmark of dependence and predicts relapse (17). It includes both affective (e.g., anxiety, sadness) and physiological (e.g., craving, hunger, concentration difficulty) components, and the current focus was on the affective aspects of withdrawal. Greater mindfulness was hypothesized to be associated with less withdrawal severity via its influence on reducing negative affect.

Mindfulness was also hypothesized to enhance cessation outcomes by increasing one's sense of agency about their ability to successfully quit smoking. Self-efficacy, a critical component of agency, has predicted relapse to smoking in numerous studies (18–20). In addition, affect regulation expectancies (another component of agency) for both smoking and nonsmoking coping predict smoking motivation, self-administration, and longitudinal changes in smoking behavior (21,22). Degree of mindfulness may enhance agency through its effects on increasing awareness of internal and external stimuli occurring in the present moment, and through increasing acceptance of distressing cognitions, emotions, perceptions, and sensations that occupy awareness (4). Thus, mindfulness may enhance flexibility in responding and ultimately expand perceived options for handling high-risk situations.

This study examined cross-sectional associations of mindfulness with demographic and smoking history variables, dependence, withdrawal severity, and agency in 158 adult smokers enrolled in a pilot smoking cessation clinical trial.

METHODS

Procedures

The current paper presents findings based on analysis of baseline data of 158 participants who were adult smokers, recruited from the Houston metropolitan area via local print media and enrolled in a randomized controlled pilot study ($N = 158$) to evaluate a mindfulness-based group therapy for nicotine dependence. In this pilot trial, participants were randomly assigned to either a mindfulness intervention or "standard of care" treatment. The mindfulness intervention included 8 weekly group therapy sessions that integrated Mindfulness-Based Stress Reduction (23) with a cognitive-behavioral relapse prevention based intervention consistent with a standard coping skills training approach (24). In this trial, after participants provided informed consent, an exhaled carbon monoxide (CO) sample was obtained and the baseline assessments were completed. Then, they were randomized. The study was approved by the Institutional Review Board of The University of Texas M. D. Anderson Cancer Center.

Participants

Participants ($N = 158$), per eligibility criteria, were tobacco cigarette smokers who had smoked at least 5 cigarettes per day for the past year, motivated to quit within next 30 days, were fluent in English, and had a home address and telephone number. Exclusion criteria included contraindication of nicotine patch use, regular use of noncigarette tobacco products, use of nicotine replacement therapies or smoking cessation pharmacotherapy other than study-provided, enrollment in another cessation program, self-reported pregnancy or lactation, psychotropic medication use, and other household members enrolled in the study. The primary reasons for exclusion from the study included a lack of motivation to quit within 30 days, regular use of tobacco products other than cigarettes, current use of nicotine replacement, and smoking <5 cigarettes per day (see Figure 1).

Measures

Demographics assessed included age, race/ethnicity, gender, marital status, educational attainment (years completed), employment status, and annual household income. Several demographic variables were categorized. Race/ethnicity was categorized as a 4-group variable (non-Latino White, non-Latino Black, Latino, and Other). Marital status, employment status, and household income level were dichotomized (married/living with partner versus not married/not living with partner; employed versus not employed; income <\$20,000 versus ≥\$20,000 per year).

Nicotine dependence severity was evaluated using the Wisconsin Inventory of Smoking Dependence Motives (WISDM-68) (16) and the Heaviness of Smoking Index (HSI) (25). The WISDM-68 is a multidimensional measure that yields an overall score and 13 subscale scores for critical dimensions of dependence. These scores have high internal consistency and reliability; and high predictive validity regarding predicting relapse (16). The WISDM-68 subscales were combined to compute Primary and Secondary Dependence Scores, with higher scores reflecting greater dependence severity (26). The HSI

FIGURE 1. Participant recruitment, screening, and study enrollment.

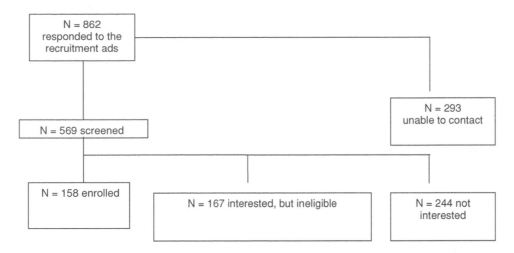

(25) is comprised of 2 items from the Fagerström Test for Nicotine Dependence (27): cigarettes per day (CPD) and time to the first cigarette after waking (TTFC). The HSI has fair internal consistency ($\alpha = .63$) (28) and the TTFC item predicts relapse (the shorter TTFC, the higher risk for relapse to smoking) (29).

Nicotine withdrawal severity was assessed prior to quitting with the Wisconsin Smoking Withdrawal Scale (WSWS) (30). The scale yields a total score and 7 subscale scores (i.e., anger, anxiety, concentration difficulty, craving, hunger, sadness, and sleep problems). All scales have excellent internal consistency and demonstrate clear increases as a function of withdrawal severity, with higher scores reflecting greater withdrawal severity (31). Because withdrawal was assessed before the quit day, smokers were not likely in physiological withdrawal at the time of the assessment; however, they were all anticipating quitting in a near future as a part of the study. Thus, the focus of the current study was on the more affective, anticipatory (e.g., anxiety, sadness) rather than physiological (e.g., craving, hunger, concentration difficulty) aspects of withdrawal.

Agency or confidence in one's ability to cope with high-risk situations without relapsing was assessed using 2 questionnaires: 1 evaluating self-efficacy (Self-Efficacy Scale (20)) and one evaluating affect regulation expectancies (Affective Information Processing Questionnaire

[AIPQ] (22)). The Self-Efficacy Scale is a 9-item measure; its total score and 3 subscale scores reflect situational categories that characterize high-risk situations: positive affect/social situations, negative affect situations, and habitual/craving situations. Higher scores reflect greater confidence in one's ability to cope in high-risk situations (20). The Self-Efficacy Scale was completed by only 116 of the 158 participants because it was inadvertently excluded from the assessment battery for the first 42 participants.

The AIPQ evaluated affect regulation expectancies by assessing responses to vignettes relating to negative affect. Participants provided ratings of the controllability of their affect in that situation (described by a vignette) by (a) smoking, and (b) means other than smoking. The AIPQ internal consistency is excellent, with both subscales predicting smoking motivation and use in laboratory settings (22), and change over time among young adults (32).

The degree of mindfulness was measured with the Kentucky Inventory of Mindfulness Skills (KIMS) and the Mindfulness Attention Awareness Scale (MAAS) (33,34). Higher scores on both measures indicate greater degree of mindfulness. The KIMS is a 39-item multidimensional measure comprising four subscales: Observing, Describing, Acting with Awareness, and Accepting without Judgment. The KIMS outcome measure is a score calculated as an average

MINDFULNESS-RELATED TREATMENTS AND ADDICTION RECOVERY

of the four subscale scores (35). Internal consistency is adequate to good with coefficient alphas ranging from .83 to .91. Test-retest reliability is adequate to good with coefficient alphas ranging from .65 to .86 and paired-sample t tests revealing no significant difference between administrations (33). Convergent validity is supported by significant positive associations between the KIMS and openness to experience ($r = .47$, $P < .01$), and the KIMS and emotional intelligence ($r = .61$, $P < .01$). Discriminant validity of the KIMS is supported by its negative associations with neuroticism ($r = -.37$, $P < .01$), thought suppression ($r = -.42$, $P < .01$), and difficulties in emotional regulation ($r = -.56$, $P < .01$) (35). The KIMS was validated in a nonclinical college student sample. The MAAS is a 15-item measure developed with a college sample and subsequently cross-validated with a nationwide sample of the U.S. adults. It has good reliability, and is associated with enhanced self-awareness and numerous other constructs indicative of well-being. It can differentiate mindfulness practitioners from nonpractitioners, and predicts self-regulation and positive emotional states (34). The mean of all items was calculated to generate the final score.

Data Analysis

Analyses were conducted using SPSS Version 16.0 statistical software. Distributional data characteristics were evaluated by conducting skewness analyses on the 31 dependent variables examined in the paper. Using the rule of thumb that a skew of less than 2 standard errors is not significant, only 7 of the 31 variables were significantly skewed (5 of 16 scales from the WISDM, the HSI, and 1 scale from the WSWS). Because the sample primarily included heavier smokers, it is not surprising that some of the measures of dependence were negatively skewed. None of the agency scales were skewed. Considering the sample size and the actual amount of skewness within these 7 variables, we elected to use multiple linear regression without correction (36). Descriptive statistics were used to describe participants' demographic and smoking history characteristics. Associations of the mindfulness measures with demographics

and smoking history were examined using Pearson product moment correlations for continuous variables, and point biserial correlations for dichotomous variables. Multiple linear regression analysis, adjusted for age, gender, race/ethnicity, educational attainment, income, and education, examined the associations of degree of mindfulness with levels of nicotine dependence, withdrawal severity, and agency. All statistical tests were 2-tailed with significance levels of $P < .05$. All individuals ($N = 158$) enrolled in the pilot study were included in the analyses. Results are presented as mean (standard deviation [SD]) unless indicated otherwise.

RESULTS

All baseline measures were completed by 158 participants, with the exception of the Self-Efficacy Scale, which was completed by 116 participants.

Participant Characteristics

Participants were 45% female; 50% were Caucasian, 34% African American, 10% Hispanic, and 6% other. The mean age was 43.8 years (11.8), and the mean years of education completed was 13.4 (2.5). Thirty-eight percent were married or cohabitating with a significant other, 57% were employed, and 34% reported their annual household income below $20,000.

They smoked an average of 20.8 (9.2) cigarettes per day, for an average of 24.8 (12.1) years. The mean baseline exhaled CO level was 21.3 (11.3) parts per million. The mean MAAS and KIMS scores were 4.2 (1.0) and 31.4 (3.8), respectively.

Associations Between Mindfulness, and Demographic/Smoking Variables

Age and years of smoking were the only demographic and smoking variables significantly associated with the degree of mindfulness; participants who were older and had longer smoking histories reported greater mindfulness as assessed by the MAAS and KIMS scores (Table 1).

TABLE 1. Pearson and Point Biserial Correlations of Demographic and Smoking-Related Variables with the Degree of Mindfulness Measures

Demographics and smoking history	MAAS score	KIMS score
Age (years)	.263***	.216**
Gender (male vs. female)	−.018	.026
Married/living with significant other (vs. not)	−.034	−.109
Education (years)	−.032	−.076
Unemployed (vs. employed)	.048	.135
Annual household income <$20,000 (vs. ≥ $20,000)	.131	.115
Cigarettes per day (number)	.039	−.019
Years smoked (years)	.186*	.167*
Carbon Monoxide (CO) level (ppm)	−.021	−.034

Note. The measures are KIMS and MAAS scores ($N = 158$); results are presented as correlation coefficients, r values.
*$P < .05$; **$P < .01$; ***$P < .001$.
MAAS = Mindfulness Attention Awareness Scale; KIMS = Kentucky Inventory of Mindfulness Skills.

Mindfulness and Dependence

As hypothesized, greater degree of mindfulness was associated with lesser nicotine dependence severity. Both the MAAS and the KIMS scores were significantly negatively associated with scores on virtually all of the WISDM-68 subscales, with the exception of Social/Environmental Goads and Tolerance subscales for the MAAS, and the Tolerance subscale for the KIMS, which were not significantly correlated with the WISDM-68 subscales (Table 2). Neither the KIMS nor the MAAS score was associated with the HSI score.

Mindfulness and Withdrawal Severity

The MAAS and KIMS scores were significantly negatively associated with all of the WSWS subscale scores, with the exception of Hunger. All significant associations were in the expected direction such that greater degree of mindfulness was associated with lesser nicotine withdrawal severity (Table 2).

Mindfulness and Agency

Degree of mindfulness was overall positively associated with self-efficacy ratings regarding one's ability to abstain from smoking in high-risk situations. The MAAS score was positively associated with the total and subscale scores of the Self-Efficacy measure. However, the KIMS score was significantly associated with only Habitual/Craving Situations of this measure. Finally, as hypothesized, the MAAS and KIMS scores were significantly associated with scores of 2 AIPQ subscales: positively with the Affect Control by Other Means score, and negatively with the Affect Control by Smoking score (Table 2).

DISCUSSION

The current findings provide the first evidence that degree of trait mindfulness is significantly associated with a combination of factors that strongly predict relapse among smokers enrolled in a cessation trial. Consistent with hypotheses, smokers reporting a higher degree of mindfulness were less nicotine dependent, experienced fewer withdrawal symptoms prior to quitting, and a stronger sense of agency regarding their ability to successfully quit smoking. Moreover, the degree of mindfulness remained significantly associated with severity of nicotine dependence and withdrawal, and level of agency, even after controlling for key demographic variables including age, gender, race/ethnicity, educational attainment, income, and marital status. This is important because each of these characteristics has been demonstrated to increase relapse vulnerability. Thus, the results suggest that the degree of mindfulness may be an important incremental predictor of vulnerability to relapse among smokers preparing to quit.

Many established predictors of the level of nicotine dependence, withdrawal, and agency (e.g., educational attainment, income, race/ethnicity, gender, years smoked) are difficult or impossible to target through a therapeutic intervention. The results indicate that levels of trait mindfulness may ultimately be useful in predicting cessation outcomes, and considerable evidence supports the efficacy of targeted interventions to enhance level of mindfulness among diverse populations and for varied outcomes (37,38). Therefore, in addition to having

TABLE 2. Means and Unstandardized Multiple Linear Regression Coefficients for Primary Study Variables

Variable	Mean (SD)	MAAS score*			KIMS Score*		
		B	SE	P	B	SE	P
WISDM-68 (n = 158), scores							
Subscales:							
Affiliative Attachment	3.6 (1.8)	−.540	.156	**.001**	−.158	.039	**<.001**
Automaticity	4.6 (1.6)	−.373	.145	**.011**	−.117	.037	**.002**
Loss of Control	5.2 (1.5)	−.358	.132	**.008**	−.080	.034	**.020**
Behavioral Choice/Melioration	3.6 (1.5)	−.504	.129	**<.001**	−.156	.032	**<.001**
Cognitive Enhancement	3.9 (1.8)	−.501	.153	**.001**	−.128	.039	**.001**
Craving	5.2 (1.4)	−.350	.126	**.006**	−.082	.032	**.012**
Cue Exposure	4.9 (1.2)	−.573	.100	**<.001**	−.117	.027	**<.001**
Negative Reinforcement	4.6 (1.5)	−.476	.122	**<.001**	−.132	.031	**<.001**
Positive Reinforcement	4.1 (1.6)	−.465	.136	**.001**	−.138	.034	**<.001**
Social/Environmental Goads	3.8 (2.0)	−.192	.165	.247	−.085	.042	**.044**
Taste and Sensory Processes	4.4 (1.5)	−.380	.130	**.004**	−.131	.032	**<.001**
Tolerance	5.2 (1.4)	−.004	.130	.976	−.043	.033	.194
Weight Control	3.2 (1.7)	−.354	.143	**.014**	−.105	.036	**.004**
Total	56.4 (14.6)	−5.07	1.25	**<.001**	−1.473	.314	**<.001**
WISDM primary	5.0 (1.2)	−.271	.108	**.013**	−.081	.027	**.004**
WISDM secondary	4.0 (1.2)	−.443	.101	**<.001**	−.128	.025	**<.001**
Heaviness of Smoking Index (HSI)	3.4 (1.4)	−.042	.030	.165	−.108	.119	.366
WSWS (n = 158), scores							
Subscales:							
Anger	1.9 (1.1)	−.524	.086	**<.001**	−.125	.022	**<.001**
Anxiety	2.1 (0.9)	−.499	.070	**<.001**	−.118	.018	**<.001**
Concentration Difficulty	1.6 (0.9)	−.485	.065	**<.001**	−.126	.017	**<.001**
Craving	2.7 (0.7)	−.150	.063	**.018**	−.033	.016	**.044**
Hunger	2.1 (0.7)	−.060	.058	.298	−.008	.015	.587
Sadness	1.6 (0.9)	−.467	.067	**<.001**	−.135	.016	**<.001**
Sleep Problems	2.1 (1.0)	−.379	.087	**<.001**	−.078	.023	**.001**
Total	2.0 (0.6)	−.366	.048	**<.001**	−.089	.012	**<.001**
Self-Efficacy/Confidence (n =116), scores							
Subscales:							
Positive Affect/Social Situations	2.5 (1.0)	.281	.098	**.005**	.030	.027	.274
Negative Affect Situations	2.2 (0.9)	.246	.091	**.008**	.039	.025	.114
Habitual/Craving Situations	2.6 (1.0)	.238	.097	**.016**	.063	.026	**.016**
Total	2.4 (0.9)	.255	.087	**.004**	.044	.024	.065
AIPQ (n = 158), subscale scores							
Affect control by other means	4.2 (1.5)	.355	.106	**.001**	.144	.025	**<.001**
Affect control by smoking	4.4 (1.2)	−.342	.126	**.007**	−.081	.032	**.014**

Note. B = unstandardized beta weight; SE = standard error; P = significance level.
*All Bs and SEs are adjusted for age, gender, educational attainment, race/ethnicity, marital status, and annual household income.
WISDM-68 = Wisconsin Inventory of Smoking Dependence Motives; WSW S = Wisconsin Smoking Withdrawal Scale; AIPQ = Affective Information Processing Questionnaire; MAAS = Mindfulness Attention Awareness Scale; KIMS = Kentucky Inventory of Mindfulness Skills.

incremental predictive utility as a marker of dependence, withdrawal severity, and agency, level of mindfulness among smokers may be malleable through intervention. We are currently conducting a large, randomized controlled trial to evaluate the efficacy of a mindfulness-based treatment for smoking cessation outcomes, and the mechanisms and effects posited to mediate the treatment's impact on tobacco abstinence.

In addition to having utility as a target for intervention, levels of trait mindfulness may be useful in matching smokers with optimal treatments. It may be that smokers who are naturally more "mindful" have an easier time quitting and may require less intensive interventions.

On the other hand, more "mindful" smokers may respond better to intensive mindfulness-based interventions because they relate better to the treatment content and are more compliant. Those with low degrees of mindfulness may also benefit from interventions teaching mindfulness skills, to increase their "mindfulness," if they agree to such therapeutic modality.

It is interesting, although not surprising, that virtually all of the WISDM-68 scales, evaluating multidimensional dependence, were negatively associated with the degree of mindfulness, whereas the HSI scores, evaluating physiological dependence, were not. It was hypothesized that mindfulness would be associated with lower levels of dependence through its effects on enhancing attentional control and positive affect, and reducing automaticity and negative affect. The WISDM-68 comprises 13 scales that assess distinct motives for smoking, 7 of which directly reflect our proposed mechanisms. Automaticity, Cue Exposure-Associative Processes, Loss of Control, and Social-Environmental Goads subscales reflect attentional control and automaticity, and Affiliative Attachment, Negative Reinforcement, and Positive Reinforcement subscales reflect affect. Thus, mindfulness appeared to be strongly and consistently associated with a broad range of motivational bases for smoking that ultimately contribute to dependence severity, but may be unrelated to purely physiological hallmarks of dependence.

A counterintuitive finding was that mindfulness was positively (although modestly) associated with years smoked, suggesting, on one hand, that mindfulness may actually inhibit one's ability to successfully quit smoking. On the other hand, years smoking and degree of mindfulness were positively associated with age. Thus, the association of mindfulness with years smoking may have simply been an artifact of these associations.

Another interesting finding was that the self-efficacy scale scores were positively and consistently associated with the MAAS, but not the KIMS scores; only 1 of the 3 self-efficacy subscales—Habitual/Craving Situations—was related to the KIMS. This lack of association was inconsistent with our hypotheses and surprising given that both the MAAS and KIMS total scores yielded a virtually identical pattern of results for all other outcomes. One possible explanation is that power may have been limited because the self-efficacy measure was not completed by all participants. It is notable that all found associations, both significant and trends, were in the expected direction. Relationships between the KIMS and the measures of self-efficacy should be examined in future research.

Several limitations should be acknowledged. First, because the data were cross-sectional, we were unable to assess whether or not degree of mindfulness was associated with cessation outcomes, or whether or not dependence severity may have mediated or moderated such potential outcomes. An additional question is whether training in mindfulness could impact levels of nicotine dependence, withdrawal, or agency, or cessation outcomes. These questions should be addressed using longitudinal data in future studies. Also, because withdrawal severity was assessed prior to cessation, participants were likely not in physiological withdrawal at the time of the assessment. However, the goal of assessing withdrawal severity at baseline was to examine associations of mindfulness with the more affective aspects of anticipated withdrawal that may emerge prior to actual cessation. Selection bias may present an additional limitation; participants were aware of the study focus on mindfulness. Therefore, they may have had higher levels of mindfulness than the general population of smokers. Our participants may not be representative of all smokers; thus, these results may not generalize beyond the current study.

Although a large proportion of smokers attempt to quit each year, few are successful (39). The majority experiences increased levels of negative affect after quitting that can persist for months, and considerable evidence indicates that difficulty with negative affect, among other factors, contributes strongly to relapse (40). Broad and consistent evidence suggests that mindfulness enhances emotional and behavioral regulation. Thus, degree of mindfulness may help reduce the distress of quitting and ultimately prevent relapse. This study provides the first preliminary evidence that degree of trait mindfulness among smokers seeking assistance with quitting is significantly associated with level of nicotine dependence, withdrawal, and agency, 3 factors that have been established as critical in predicting vulnerability to relapse. Taken together, the results indicate that degree of trait mindfulness is associated with several factors known to predict smoking cessation and relapse. Future research should investigate potential associations of levels of trait mindfulness with cessation outcomes, as well as the efficacy and effectiveness of smoking cessation interventions intended to enhance levels of mindfulness.

REFERENCES

1. Mokdad AH, Marks JS, Stroup DF, Gerberding JL. Actual causes of death in the United States, 2000. *JAMA.* 2004;291:1238–1245.

2. Wetter DW, Fiore MC, Baker TB, Young TB. Tobacco withdrawal and nicotine replacement influence objective measures of sleep. *J Consult Clin Psychol.* 1995;63:658–667.

3. Teasdale JD. The relationship between cognition and emotion: the mind-in-place in mood disorders. In: Clark DM, Fairburn CG, eds. *Science and Practice of Cognitive Behaviour Therapy.* Oxford: Oxford University Press; 1997:67–93.

4. Roemer L, Orsillo SM. Mindfulness: a promising intervention strategy in need of further study. *Clin Psychol Sci Pract.* 2003;10:172–178.

5. Davis JM, Fleming MF, Bonus KA, Baker TB. A pilot study on mindfulness based stress reduction for smokers. *BMC Comple Altern Med.* 2007;7:2.

6. Gifford EV, Kohlenberg BS, Hayes SC, Antonuccio DO, Piasecki MM, Rasmussen-Hall M, Palm KM. Acceptance-based treatment for smoking cessation. *Behav Ther.* 2004;35:689–705.

7. Altner N. Mindfulness practice and smoking cessation: the Essen Hospital Smoking Cessation Study (EASY). *J Meditat Meditat Res.* 2002;1:9–18.

8. Zgierska A, Rabago D, Zuelsdorff M, Coe C, Miller M, Fleming M. Mindfulness meditation for alcohol relapse prevention: a feasibility pilot study. *J Addict Med.* 2008;2:165–173.

9. Breslau N, Johnson EO. Predicting smoking cessation and major depression in nicotine-dependent smokers. *Am J Public Health* 2000;90:1122–1127.

10. Davidson RJ, Kabat-Zinn J, Schumacher J, Rosenkranz M, Muller D, Santorelli SF, Urbanowski F, Harrington A, Bonus K, Sheridan JF. Alterations in brain and immune function produced by mindfulness meditation. *Psychosom Med.* 2003;65:564–570.

11. Brown KW, Ryan RM. The benefits of being present: mindfulness and its role in psychological well-being. *Journal of personality and social psychology.* 2003;84:822–848.

12. Kenford SL, Smith SS, Wetter DW, Jorenby DE, Fiore MC, Baker TB. Predicting relapse back to smoking: contrasting affective and physical models of dependence. *J Consult Clin Psychol.* 2002;70:216–227.

13. Baker TB, Piper ME, McCarthy DE, Majeskie MR, Fiore MC. Addiction motivation reformulated: an affective processing model of negative reinforcement. *Psychol Rev.* 2004;111:33–51.

14. Teasdale JD, Moore RG, Hayhurst H, Pope M, Williams S, Segal ZV. Metacognitive awareness and prevention of relapse in depression: empirical evidence. *J Consult Clin Psychol.* 2002;70:275–287.

15. Tiffany ST. A cognitive model of drug urges and drug-use behavior: role of automatic and nonautomatic processes. *Psychol Rev.* 1990;97:147–168.

16. Piper ME, Piasecki TM, Federman EB, Bolt DM, Smith SS, Fiore MC, Baker TB. A multiple motives approach to tobacco dependence: the Wisconsin Inventory of Smoking Dependence Motives (WISDM-68). *J Consult Clin Psychol.* 2004;72:139–154.

17. Piasecki TM, Kenford SL, Smith SS, Fiore MC, Baker TB. Listening to nicotine: negative affect and the smoking withdrawal conundrum. *Psychol Sci.* 1997;8:184–189.

18. Baer JS, Holt CS, Lichtenstein E. Self-efficacy and smoking reexamined: construct validity and clinical utility. *J Consult Clin Psychol.* 1986;54:846–852.

19. McIntyre KO, Lichtenstein E, Mermelstein RJ. Self-efficacy and relapse in smoking cessation: a replication and extension. *J Consult Clin Psychol.* 1983;51:632–633.

20. Velicer WF, Diclemente CC, Rossi JS, Prochaska JO. Relapse situations and self-efficacy: an integrative model. *Addict Behav.* 1990;15:271–283.

21. Brandon TH, Wetter DW, Baker TB. Affect, expectancies, urges, and smoking: do they conform to models of drug motivation and relapse? *Exp Clin Psychopharmacol.* 1996;41:29–36.

22. Wetter DW, Brandon TH, Baker TB. The relation of affective processing measures and smoking motivation indices among college-age smokers. *Adv Behav Res Ther.* 1992;14:169–193.

23. Kabat-Zinn J. *Full Catastrophe Living: Using the Wisdom of Your Body and Mind to Face Stress, Pain, and Illness.* New York: Dell; 1990.

24. Fiore MC, Bailey WC, Cohen SJ, Dorfman SF, Goldstein MG, Gritz ER, et al. *Treating Tobacco Use and Dependence: Clinical Practice Guideline.* Rockville, MD: U.S. Department of Health and Human Services (USDHHS), Public Health Service (PHS); 2000. Report No.: 1-58763-007-9.

25. Kozlowski LT, Porter CQ, Orleans CT, Pope MA, Heatherton T. Predicting smoking cessation with self-reported measures of nicotine dependence: FTQ, FTND, and HSI. *Drug Alcohol Depend.* 1994;34:211–216.

26. Piper ME, Bolt DM, Kim SY, Japuntich SJ, Smith SS, Niederdeppe J, Cannon DS, Baker TB. Refining the tobacco dependence phenotype using the Wisconsin Inventory of Smoking Dependence Motives. *J Abnorm Psychol.* 2008;117:747–761.

27. Heatherton TF, Kozlowski LT, Frecker RC, Fagerstrom KO. The Fagerstrom Test for Nicotine Dependence: a revision of the Fagerstrom Tolerance Questionnaire. *Br J Addict.* 1991;86:1119–1127.

28. Etter JF. A comparison of the content-, construct- and predictive validity of the cigarette dependence scale and the Fagerstrom test for nicotine dependence. *Drug Alcohol Depend.* 2005;77:259–268.

29. Baker TB, Piper ME, McCarthy DE, Bolt DM, Smith SS, Kim SY, Colby S, Conti D, Giovino GA, Hatsukami D, Hyland A, Krishnan-Sarin S, Niaura R, Perkins KA, Toll BA. Time to first cigarette in the morning as an index of ability to quit smoking: implications for nicotine dependence. *Nicotine Tob Res.* 2007;9(Suppl 4):S555–S570.

30. Welsch SK, Smith SS, Wetter DW, Jorenby DE, Fiore MC, Baker TB. Development and validation of the Wisconsin Smoking Withdrawal Scale. *Exp Clin Psychopharmacol.* 1999;7:354–361.

31. Wetter DW, Carmack CL, Anderson CB, Moore CA, De Moor CA, Cinciripini PM, Hirshkowitz M. Tobacco withdrawal signs and symptoms among women with and without a history of depression. *Exp Clin Psychopharmacol.* 2000;8:88–96.

32. Wetter DW, Kenford SL, Welsch SK, Smith SS, Fouladi RT, Fiore MC, Baker TB. Prevalence and predictors of transitions in smoking behavior among college students. *Health Psychol.* 2004;23:168–177.

33. Baer RA, Smith GT, Allen KB. Assessment of mindfulness by self-report: the Kentucky inventory of mindfulness skills. *Assessment* 2004;11:191–206.

34. Brown KW, Ryan RM. The benefits of being present: mindfulness and its role in psychological well-being. *J Pers Soc Psychol.* 2003;84:822–848.

35. Baer RA, Smith GT, Hopkins J, Krietemeyer J, Toney L. Using self-report assessment methods to explore facets of mindfulness. *Assessment* 2006;13:27–45.

36. Tabachnick BG, Fidell LS. *Using Multivariate Statistics.* 3rd ed. New York: Harper Collins; 1996.

37. Ma HS, Teasdale JD. Mindfulness-based cognitive therapy for depression: replication and exploration of differential relapse prevention effects. *J Consult Clin Psychol.* 2004;72:31–40.

38. Kabat-Zinn J, Wheeler E, Light T, Skillings A, Scharf MJ, Cropley TG, Hosmer D, Bernhard JD. Influence of a mindfulness meditation-based stress reduction intervention on rates of skin clearing in patients with moderate to severe psoriasis undergoing phototherapy (UVB) and photochemotherapy (PUVA). *Psychosom Med.* 1998;60:625–632.

39. CDC. Cigarette smoking among adults—United States, 1994. *MMWR Morb Mort Wkly Rep.* 1996;27:588–590.

40. Hughes JR. The future of smoking cessation therapy in the United States. *Addiction* 1996;91:1797–1802.

Associations Between Mindfulness and Implicit Cognition and Self-Reported Affect

Andrew J. Waters, PhD
Lorraine R. Reitzel, PhD
Paul Cinciripini, PhD
Yisheng Li, PhD
Marianne T. Marcus, EdD, RN
Jennifer Irvin Vidrine, PhD
David W. Wetter, PhD

ABSTRACT. Theory suggests that mindful individuals exhibit enhanced attentional processing (e.g., attentional control) and that they maintain a detached perspective to problematic stimuli. For smokers, smoking and affective stimuli are problematic stimuli when they try to quit. In this cross-sectional study, smokers ($n = 158$) completed 3 modified Stroop tasks (to assess attentional control), 3 Implicit Association Tests (IATs; to assess detached perspective), and a battery of self-report assessments. Degree of mindfulness was negatively associated ($P < .05$) with self-reported negative affect, perceived stress, and depressive symptom severity, and positively associated ($P < .05$) with positive affect. Degree of mindfulness was not associated with the ability to disengage attention from smoking or affective stimuli. On the depression IAT, more mindful participants exhibited a more negative IAT effect, suggesting that they may have developed a detached perspective to depression-related stimuli. Theoretical and clinical implications of the data are discussed.

Andrew J. Waters is affiliated with the Department of Medical and Clinical Psychology, Uniformed Services University of the Health Sciences, Bethesda, Maryland, USA.

Lorraine R. Reitzel, Jennifer Irvin Vidrine, and David W. Wetter are affiliated with the Department of Health Disparities Research, The University of Texas M. D. Anderson Cancer Center, Houston, Texas, USA.

Paul Cinciripini is affiliated with the Department of Behavioral Science, The University of Texas M. D. Anderson Cancer Center, Houston, Texas, USA.

Yisheng Li is affiliated with the Department of Biostatistics, The University of Texas M. D. Anderson Cancer Center, Houston, Texas, USA.

Marianne T. Marcus is affiliated with the Center for Substance Abuse Prevention, Education and Research, School of Nursing, University of Texas Health Science Center, Houston, Texas, USA.

This research and preparation of this article were supported by grants from the National Institute on Drug Abuse R01 DA018875 (D.W.W.), the Centers for Disease Control and Prevention K01 DP00008 (J.I.V.) and K01 DP001120 (L.R.R.).

INTRODUCTION

Theoretical analyses and empirical data suggest that mindfulness-based interventions may be a useful treatment for substance use disorders, including tobacco dependence (1–5). Mindfulness has been defined as "paying attention in a particular way: on purpose, in the present moment, and non-judgmentally" (6). Shapiro and colleagues identified 3 axioms of mindfulness: "Intention," "Attention," and "Attitude" (7). Intention refers to the reasons why an individual chooses to practice mindfulness. Attention refers to the process by which an individual observes his or her moment-to-moment conscious experiences. Attitude refers to how an individual relates to or interprets the content of conscious experience. Similarly, Bishop and colleagues describe 2 components: increased attention to immediate conscious experience, and the development of an attitude of openness and acceptance toward that conscious experience (8). Thus, there is agreement among theorists that acquiring mindfulness skills may result in changes in cognitive processes related to "Attention" and "Attitude."

The "Attention" axiom itself has 2 subcomponents, "mindful awareness" and "attentional control." Mindful awareness refers to the ability to attend to the contents of consciousness on a moment-by-moment basis. Perhaps as a consequence of extensive practice at manipulating the spotlight of attention (9), mindfulness may improve other components of attention, such as sustained attention, attention switching, and inhibition of elaborative processing ("attentional control") (7,8,10). For example, in depressive disorders, enhanced attentional control engendered by mindfulness may allow attention to be redirected from depressive or anxious rumination back to the experience of the present moment with resulting improvement in clinical outcomes (11,12). Moreover, there is evidence that improvement in the degree of mindfulness can enhance certain attentional processes (10,13). One may therefore view the development of mindfulness skills as a form of attention retraining.

However, mindfulness can be more than just attention retraining. Mindfulness practice teaches an individual to process the contents of conscious awareness in a nonjudgmental manner ("Attitude" component), and to experience cognitions and emotions as mental events in a broader context of awareness (12). Hayes and colleagues conceptualize the shift from "self as content" (the self is an object in consciousness) to "self as context" (the self is observing the objects in consciousness and is not the object itself) (14). That is, individuals can allow distressing thoughts and feelings to occupy awareness, without necessarily trying to change them and without becoming engaged in their content. Thus, in a context of mindfulness, thoughts and feelings can be viewed simply as passing mental events that may or may not reflect reality. Ultimately, an individual realizes that "this depression is not me" and "these thoughts are not me."

In the current study, we examined the associations between questionnaire-assessed mindfulness and affect/cognition in smokers enrolled in a smoking cessation study. The rationale for the focus on self-reported affect is twofold: Self-reported affect is associated with both mindfulness (e.g., 15,16) and smoking cessation (e.g., 17,18). The rationale for the focus on attention and attitude is likewise twofold. As noted above, mindfulness should be associated with the ability to disengage attention from smoking or affective stimuli, and to maintain a detached perspective to those stimuli. In addition, improved attention (19) and a detached attitude may assist smokers trying to quit. Stated simply, an effect of mindfulness training on smoking cessation might be mediated through an effect on affect/cognition. To gather initial data on this issue, we examined the association between questionnaire-assessed mindfulness and affect/cognition in smokers.

To summarize, in this cross-sectional study we examined the following hypotheses. First, consistent with the extant literature and theory (15), we hypothesized that mindfulness should be positively associated with positive affect, and negatively associated with negative affect, stress, and depression. Second, we hypothesized that mindfulness should be associated with reduced identification with problematic stimuli. Third, we hypothesized that mindfulness should be associated with an enhanced ability to disengage attention from problematic stimuli.

METHODS

Main Study

The current manuscript presents an analysis of the baseline data of 158 adult smokers, recruited from the Houston metropolitan area, who were enrolled in a randomized controlled pilot study to evaluate a mindfulness-based group therapy treatment for nicotine dependence. Details of study procedures, including inclusion and exclusion criteria, are described in detail elsewhere (20). The study was approved by the Institutional Review Board of The University of Texas M. D. Anderson Cancer Center.

Participants

Participants were 158 adult smokers who reported smoking 5+ cigarettes a day for the past year, and that they were motivated to quit smoking within the next 30 days.

Procedures

Interested prospective subjects ($N = 569$) completed an initial telephone interview during which their eligibility was assessed. Eligible individuals were invited to attend an in-person informational and enrollment meeting, which occurred on average 7.4 (SD = 4.2) days after the telephone interview. Then, enrolled subjects ($N = 158$) completed their baseline assessments, which included the Stroop tasks and IATs (completed in that order) and computer-administered questionnaires.

Measures

After verbal consent was obtained, demographic assessments and the Center of Epidemiologic Studies Depression Scale (CESD) (21) were administered at the telephone interview. Other assessments were administered at the baseline visit.

Questionnaire Measures

Degree of mindfulness was assessed using the 15-item Mindfulness Attention Awareness Scale (MAAS) and the 39-item Kentucky Inventory of Mindfulness Skills (KIMS). MAAS scores (mean score on the 15 items) have been shown to correlate with level of well-being, to differentiate mindfulness practitioners from nonpractitioners, and to predict self-regulation and positive emotional states (15). The KIMS is a multidimensional questionnaire that yields 4 scales: Observing, Describing, Acting with Awareness, and Accepting without Judgment. Internal consistency and test-retest reliability of the KIMS is good, as is convergent and discriminant validity (22). "Observing" most closely captures the process by which attention is deliberatively focused on the contents of consciousness ("mindful awareness"). "Describing" assesses the tendency to apply verbal labels to the contents of conscious experience. "Acting with Awareness" assesses the ability to engage undivided attention in a current task. "Accepting without Judgment" best captures the "Attitude" component (detached perspective).

Depressive symptom severity was assessed with the CESD (21), which has good psychometric properties and has been widely used in smoking cessation research (e.g., 23).

Positive and negative affect was evaluated using the Positive and Negative Affect Scale (PANAS), which is comprised of 2 mood scales: Positive (PA) and Negative (NA) Affect (24). The PANAS-NA scores have been reported to be among the best predictors of tobacco relapse (17).

Stress symptom severity was evaluated using the Perceived Stress Scale (PSS), a 4-item measure designed to assess the degree to which respondents have experienced stress (25). The PSS total score is predictive of relapse (26).

Cognitive Assessments

We assessed "Attention" and "Attitude" using implicit cognitive assessments. Recent theory and empirical research in the field of addiction have emphasized the utility of implicit cognitive assessments (27, 28). We administered the Implicit Association Test (IAT) (assessment of "Attitude") and the modified Stroop task (assessment of "Attention"). Both tasks have been widely used to study addiction (e.g., 29,30), and psychopathology (e.g., 31,32); the IAT has also been used to study mindfulness (15,33). We focused on responses to affective and smoking-related stimuli, which are problematic stimuli for smokers trying to quit (e.g., 18,19). Three IATs and 3 modified Stroop tasks were administered on a desktop computer using E-prime software (version 1.1) (34). Order of completion of the IATs was counterbalanced across participants; the same was true for the modified Stroop tasks. Each IAT and Stroop task took around 5 and 2 minutes to complete, respectively.

IAT. On the IAT, participants were asked to respond rapidly by pressing a certain keyboard key for items representing 2 concepts (e.g., depressed + me), and with a different key for items from 2 other concepts (e.g., not depressed + not me) (Task 1). In Task 2, the assignment of one concept was switched, such that, for example, "not depressed" + "me" shared a common key-response, and "depressed" + "not me" shared the other response. The idea underlying the IAT is that it is easier to perform the IAT when the 2 concepts are strongly associated in memory than when the 2 concepts are unrelated (35). The critical outcome measure (the IAT effect) is the difference in reaction times (RTs) on Task 1 versus Task 2. The IAT effect is considered an index of the relative strength of mental associations. In the example above, it indicates whether associations are stronger between depressed and me, and not depressed and not me, than between not depressed and me, and depressed and not me.

Each participant completed a smoking IAT (smoking/not smoking, me/not me), an anxiety IAT (anxious/not anxious, me/not me), and a depression IAT (depressed/not depressed, me/not me). Lower (more negative) scores on these IATs (e.g., faster responses when "depression" is paired with "not me" compared to when "depression" is paired with "me") are interpreted as indicating a more detached perspective to depression, anxiety or smoking stimuli.

Each IAT consisted of 7 blocks: (1) Practice of categorization for the target concept (e.g., depressed/not depressed); (2) Practice of categorization for me/not me; (3) First block of combined categorization task (Task 1); (4) Second block for Task 1; (5) Practice of categorization for the target concept but with the response keys reversed from the assignment in (1) (not depressed/depressed); (6) First block of alternative combined categorization task (Task 2); (7) Second block for Task 2. The order in which participants performed the combined categorization blocks (i.e., 3–4 and 6–7) was counterbalanced across participants. Blocks 1, 2, and 3 each had 20 trials, and blocks 4, 5, 6, and 7 each had 40 trials.

For the smoking IAT, we used smoking and nonsmoking pictures from a previous study (30). For the anxiety IAT, the anxious words were jittery, nervous, jumpy, troubled, uptight, stressed, tense, strained, fidgety, and irritable. The not anxious words were calm, cool, relaxed, unconcerned, unworried, untroubled, carefree, restful, composed, and comfortable. For the depression IAT, the depressed words were sad, lonely, hopeless, guilty, unhappy, discouraged, gloomy, low, depressed, and failure. The not depressed words were content, joyful, happy, cheerful, pleased, fun, merry, funny, excited, and positive. Me/not me words were derived from previous IAT research (15). "Me" words included I, me, and mine. "Not me" words included they, them, and other. The same "me/not me" words were used in all IATs.

Procedure. On each trial, a stimulus (word or picture) was presented in the center of a computer monitor. On the top of the screen were labels (on each side of the screen) to remind participants of the categories assigned to each key for the current task. Participants responded to the categorization task by pressing either an "L" key or the "R" key on the keyboard as quickly as possible (see (36) for further details of procedures).

Scoring. We used a currently recommended scoring algorithm (see 37) that involves dividing the IAT effect (difference in mean RTs on Tasks 1 and 2) by the pooled standard deviation of RTs. This algorithm also eliminates assessments on which a participant had RTs of <300 ms on more than 10% of trials (6, 9, and 7 assessments for the smoking, anxiety, and depression IATs, respectively), and RTs > 10,000 ms. RTs on incorrect responses were replaced by the block mean (correct responses) plus 600 ms. For comparability with other research, we also elected to present the IAT effect in milliseconds. Due to experimenter error, computer error, or subject circumstances, 11 subjects did not complete the IATs.

Modified Stroop Task

Participants completed 3 40-trial Stroop tasks: 1 containing smoking (e.g., cigarette) and neutral words (e.g., tablespoon); 1 containing anxiety (e.g., stressed) and neutral words; and 1 containing depression (e.g., sad) and neutral words. For all tasks, a mixed randomized format was used to examine the impact of the smoking or affective words on RTs on the subsequent trial (38–40). The carry-over effect (or "slow" Stroop effect) (38) may index the degree of difficulty in disengaging attention from the target stimulus (smoking or affective words).

Participants were instructed that words written in different colors will be presented on the screen, one after the other, and that their task was to indicate as rapidly and as accurately as possible which color the word was written in, by pressing 1 of 3 colored buttons on a keyboard. They were instructed to ignore the meaning of the word itself and to respond just to the color (see 19 for details).

The smoking words were tobacco, cigarette, smoke, craving, urge, ashtray, lighter, puff, drag, and nicotine. The depression and anxiety words were the same as those used in the respective IATs. There were 10 neutral words (household features) in each Stroop task; different neutral words were used in each Stroop task. The smoking, depression, and anxiety words did not differ in length or frequency from their respective neutral words using established norms (41).

Scoring. RTs < 100 ms and RTs on incorrect responses were excluded from analyses (2.85% of data); data from 1 subject were excluded because the subject's error rate was >33%. The carry-over effect was computed from the difference in RTs on trials after smoking words (or after depression or anxiety words) versus trials after neutral words. Due to experimenter error, computer error, or subject circumstances, 5 subjects did not complete the Stroop tasks.

Data Analysis Plan

One hundred fifty-eight subjects were included in the analyses. Analyses were conducted using SAS version 9.1. Visual inspection of the data revealed that IAT and Stroop effects appeared to be normally distributed. Scores on the mindfulness questionnaires, the PANAS-PA, and the PSS also appeared normally distributed; scores on the PANAS-NA and CESD appeared to be positively skewed. Descriptive statistics were used to describe participants' demographic and smoking history characteristics, self-reported affect, perceived stress, depressive symptom severity, IAT effects, and carry-over effects. Results are presented as mean (standard deviation [SD]) unless otherwise specified.

All correlational analyses were conducted using Pearson product moment correlations. Pearson's r has been shown to be robust to violations in normality (42). Analyses on IAT effects used the D score. All statistical tests were 2-tailed. Alpha was set to .05.

RESULTS

Participants' ($N = 158$) average age was 43.8 (11.8) years. Fifty-five percent were male. Participants smoked an average of 20.8 (9.2) cigarettes per day for an average of 24.8 (12.1) years. Details of participants' demographics are described elsewhere (20).

Descriptive Statistics

On the IAT, participants exhibited a robust implicit self-identification with smoking (versus not smoking; $t = 3.14$, $df = 140$, $P < .01$), not anxious (versus anxious; $t = -9.51$, $df = 137$, $P < .01$), and not depressed (versus depressed; $t = -10.6$, $df = 139$, $P < .01$) (Table 1).

On the modified Stroop task, participants were slower to perform the correct color classifications on words that followed: smoking words (versus neutral words; $t = 2.82$, $df = 151$, $P < .01$), and depression words (versus neutral words; $t = 4.33$, $df = 151$, $P < .01$); they also tended to be slower on words that followed anxiety words (versus neutral words; $t = 1.86$, $df = 151$, $P = .06$) (Table 1).

TABLE 1. Descriptive Statistics for Study Measures

Measure	N	M	SD
MAAS	158	4.2	1.0
KIMS-Observing	158	37.0	7.0
KIMS-Describing	158	28.1	5.6
KIMS-Acting with Awareness	158	31.3	5.4
KIMS-Accepting	158	29.3	6.4
PANAS-PA	158	32.4	9.0
PANAS-NA	158	20.9	8.9
PSS	158	6.6	3.1
CESD	158	17.1	12.9
Smoking IAT (ms)	141	102	389
Anxiety IAT (ms)	138	−279	347
Depression IAT (ms)	140	−340	383
Smoking IAT (D score)	141	0.12	0.59
Anxiety IAT (D score)	138	−0.53	0.52
Depression IAT (D score)	140	−0.57	0.50
Smoking Stroop (ms)	152	19.2	83.8
Anxiety Stroop (ms)	152	12.1	80.1
Depression Stroop (ms)	152	23.8	67.7

Note. Key: MAAS = Mindfulness Attention Awareness Scale; KIMS = Kentucky Inventory of Mindfulness Skills; PANAS-NA = Negative affect scale of the Positive and Negative Affect Scale; PANAS-PA = Positive affect scale of the Positive and Negative Affect Scale; PSS = Perceived Stress Scale; CESD = Center of Epidemiologic Studies Depression Scale; IAT = Implicit Association Test; D score = method of scoring IAT (see text); N = number of participants contributing data on each measure. Data shown for Stroop tasks shows carry-over effect in ms (see text for details).

Association Between Mindfulness and Self-Reported Affect

As expected, the degree of mindfulness, assessed by MAAS, was negatively correlated ($P < .05$) with symptom severity of depression, negative affect, and stress, and positively correlated ($P < .05$) with positive affect (Table 2).

On the KIMS mindfulness questionnaire, the scores of the Describing, Acting with Awareness, and Accepting scales, but not of the Observing scale, were correlated ($P < .05$) with symptom severity of depression, negative affect, and stress in the expected direction. All KIMS scales were correlated ($P < .05$) with positive affect in the expected direction (Table 2).

Association Between Mindfulness and Implicit Measures

MAAS-assessed degree of mindfulness was negatively correlated ($P < .05$) with the depression IAT, but not the anxiety IAT or the smoking IAT (Table 2); higher MAAS scores were associated with a lower (more negative) depression IAT effect (Figure 1). That is, more mindful participants (higher MAAS score) found it easier to perform the classification task when depression was paired with not me compared to when depression was paired with me. Table 2 shows that Describing and Accepting (but not Observing or Acting with Awareness) were negatively correlated ($P < .05$) with the depression IAT.

There were no significant correlations between the mindfulness measures and the carry-over effects on the modified Stroop task (Table 2).

TABLE 2. Pearson's Correlation Coefficients (*r*) Between Mindfulness, Implicit Measures, and Self-Reported Affect

	Implicit						Self-Report			
	Smoking IAT	Anxiety IAT	Depression IAT	Smoking carry-over	Anxiety carry-over	Depression carry-over	PANAS-PA	PANAS-NA	PSS	CESD
MAAS	.00	−.14	**−.27****	.15	.01	.07	**.28****	**−.44****	**−.45****	**−.33****
KIMS-Observing	.07	−.07	.05	−.04	−.02	.06	**.31****	.07	−.01	−.01
KIMS-Describing	−.01	−.03	**−.23****	−.09	−.00	.09	**.50****	**−.25****	**−.41****	**−.25****
KIMS-Acting with Awareness	−.06	−.16	−.14	.11	−.05	.05	**.18***	**−.41****	**−.35****	**−.27****
KIMS-Accepting	−.10	−.12	**−.18***	.09	−.04	.11	**.28****	**−.54****	**−.45****	**−.35****

Note. Key: MAAS = Mindfulness Attention Awareness Scale; KIMS = Kentucky Inventory of Mindfulness Skills; PANAS-NA = Negative affect scale of the Positive and Negative Affect Scale; PANAS-PA = Positive affect scale of the Positive and Negative Affect Scale; PSS = Perceived Stress Scale; CESD = Center of Epidemiologic Studies Depression Scale; IAT = Implicit Association Test. Ns are 141 (smoking IAT), 138 (anxiety IAT), 140 (depression IAT), 152 (Carry-over effects), and 158 (all other variables). On the MAAS and the KIMS, higher scores indicate more mindfulness. Significant correlations are in bold.
*$P < .05$; **$P < .01$.

FIGURE 1. Scatterplot of relationship between MAAS-assessed degree of mindfulness (mean item score) and the IAT effect (in ms) on the depression IAT. The best-fit regression line is shown for illustrative purposes. Positive IAT values reflect the extent to which participants are faster to perform the classification task when depression is paired with me (versus not me). Negative IAT values reflect the extent to which participants are slower to perform the classification task when depression is paired with me (versus not me). MAAS = Mindfulness Attention Awareness Scale; IAT = Implicit Association Test.

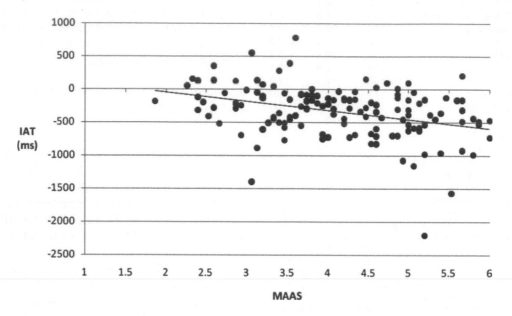

DISCUSSION

This cross-sectional study of 158 smokers examined the associations between questionnaire-assessed mindfulness and affect/cognition. This is one of a few studies to apply the methods of implicit cognition to the study of mindfulness (15,33). It yielded several key findings. First, consistent with previous data (15), the degree of mindfulness was robustly associated with self-reported affect, stress, and depressive symptom severity. Second, the degree of mindfulness was negatively associated with implicit self-identification with depression (but not anxiety or smoking). Third, there was no evidence that mindfulness was associated with the ability to disengage attention from problematic stimuli.

Perhaps the most interesting finding of the study was the association between questionnaire-assessed mindfulness and the depression IAT effect. Confidence in the reliability of this observed association is bolstered by the

fact that it was observed for both the MAAS questionnaire and (two) KIMS scales, and by the fact that there was a robust correlation between the degree of mindfulness and the depression IAT effect assessed on participants' quit day (not reported in paper). Following the logic of the IAT (35), the data indicate that greater mindfulness is associated with weaker automatic mental associations between "depressed" and "me" concepts and/or stronger automatic mental associations between "depressed" and "not me" concepts.[1] Interestingly, the association between questionnaire-assessed mindfulness and the depression IAT effect seemed more evident in the Attitude (detached perspective) component of mindfulness on the KIMS questionnaire (Describing and Accepting without Judgment).

Contrary to the study hypotheses, a correlation between mindfulness and the IAT effect was not observed for anxiety or smoking concepts. The reason for these null associations is not clear. Regarding the latter, it is possible that mindfulness in unselected participants (like those in the current study) targets affective rather than smoking stimuli.

Participants exhibited robust carry-over effects on all 3 modified Stroop tasks. Consistent with previous data, this suggests that they experienced difficulty disengaging attention from the salient smoking and affective words (39). However, we did not find any relationship between questionnaire-assessed degree of mindfulness and the carry-over effects. The meaning of this finding is not clear. In previous studies where an effect of mindfulness-based training on attention had been reported, participants had received an intensive mindfulness-based intervention (10, 13). In addition, an effect of mindfulness might be observed on alternative measures of attentional disengagement, such as those assessed by the visual probe task (43).

Limitations

The main limitation of the study is that it was restricted to a cross-sectional analysis of baseline data. Thus, the casual relationships linking mindfulness, implicit cognition, and well-being remain uncertain. In addition, we administered only a single measure of attention. The study was also limited to heavy adult smokers who wished to quit. We do not know whether our findings would generalize to other populations of smokers, or other substances abusers.

Strengths

We included a comprehensive battery of self-report affect and mindfulness measures. In addition, our assessment strategy was guided by a conceptual analysis of the cognitive processes underlying mindfulness.

To our knowledge, this study is the first to evaluate the association between mindfulness and affect/cognition in smokers. The data are potentially theoretically and clinically important. Theoretically, the data suggest that an association between mindfulness and cognition in smokers is most apparent on a measure that assesses a detached perspective to depression stimuli. It is possible that this cognitive assessment is the most sensitive to mindfulness training and captures a fundamental feature of mindfulness. Clinically, it is possible that

performance on the depression IAT may help to identify smokers who do not possess a detached perspective; these smokers may therefore benefit the most from a mindfulness-based treatment that promotes such a perspective. Further research is required to more comprehensively characterize the relationships between mindfulness training, affect/cognition, and smoking cessation.

NOTE

1. According to the logic of the IAT (35), this interpretation requires that mindfulness is not associated with correspondingly weaker associations between "not depressed" and "not me," and/or stronger associations between "not depressed" and "me." Given that mindfulness-based therapies most commonly target negative emotions (e.g., depression), we assume that the detached perspective component of mindfulness is more readily applied to negative (e.g., depressed) than positive cognitions/absence of negative cognitions (e.g., not depressed).

REFERENCES

1. Davis JM, Fleming MF, Bonus KA, Baker TB. A pilot study on mindfulness based stress reduction for smokers. *BMC Comple Altern Med.* 2007; 7:2 doi:10.1186/1472-6882-7-2.

2. Gifford EV, Kohlenberg BS, Hayes SC, Antonuccio DO, Piasecki MM, Rasmussen-Hall ML, Palm KM. Acceptance-based treatment for smoking cessation. *Behav Ther.* 2004;35:689–705.

3. Marlatt GA, Witkiewitz K, Dillworth TM, Bowen SW, Parks GA, MacPherson LM, Lonczak HS, Larimer ME, Simpson T, Blume AW, Crutcher R. Vipassana meditation as a treatment for alcohol and drug use disorders. In: Hayes SC, Linehan MM, Follette VM, eds. *Mindfulness and Acceptance: Expanding the Cognitive-Behavioral Tradition.* New York: Guildford Press; 2004:261–287.

4. Witkiewitz K, Marlatt GA, Walker D. Mindfulness-based relapse prevention for alcohol and substance use disorders: the meditative tortoise wins the race. *J Cogn Psychother.* 2006;19:211–228.

5. Zgierska A, Rabago D, Zuelsdorff M, Coe C, Miller M, Fleming M. Mindfulness meditation for alcohol relapse prevention: a feasibility pilot study. *J Addict Med.* 2008;2:165–173.

6. Kabat-Zinn J. *Wherever You Go, There You Are: Mindfulness Meditation in Everyday Life.* New York: Hyperion; 1994.

7. Shapiro SL, Carlson LE, Astin JA, Freedman B. Mechanisms of mindfulness. *J Clin Psychol.* 2006;62: 373–386.

8. Bishop SR, Lau M, Shapiro S, Carlson L, Anderson NC, Carmody J, Segal ZV, Abbey S, Speca M, Velting D, Devins G. Mindfulness: a proposed operational definition. *Clin Psychol Sci Pract.* 2004;11:230–241.

9. Posner MI, Petersen SE. The attention system of the human brain. *Annu Rev Neurosci.* 1990;13:25–42.

10. Chambers R, Chuen Yee Lo B, Allen NB. The impact of intensive mindfulness training on attentional control, cognitive style, and affect. *Cogn Ther Res.* 2008;32:303–322.

11. Teasdale JD, Segal Z, Williams JMG. How does cognitive therapy prevent depressive relapse and why should attentional control (mindfulness) training help? *Behav Res Ther.* 1995;33:25–39.

12. Teasdale JD, Moore RG, Hayhurst H, Pope M, Williams S, Segal ZV. Metacognitive awareness and prevention of relapse in depression: empirical evidence. *Journal of Consulting and Clinical Psychology,* 2002;70:275–287.

13. Slagter HA, Lutz A, Greischar LL, Francis AD, Nieuwenhuis S, Davis JM, Davidson RJ. Mental training affects distribution of limited brain resources. *PLoS Biol.* 2007;5:e138.

14. Hayes SC, Strosahl K, Wilson KG. *Acceptance and Commitment Therapy: An Experiential Approach to Behavior Change.* New York: Guilford Press; 1999.

15. Brown K, Ryan R. The benefits of being present: mindfulness and Its role in psychological well-being. *J Person Soc Psychol.* 2003;84: 822–848.

16. Baer RA, Smith GT, Lykins E, Button D, Krietmeyer J, Sauer S, Walsh E, Duggan D, Williams JMG. Construct validity of the five facet mindfulness questionnaire in meditating and non-meditating samples. *Assessment.* 2008;15:329–342.

17. Wetter DW, Kenford SL, Smith SS, Fiore MC, Jorenby DE, Baker TB. Gender differences in smoking cessation. *J Consult Clin Psychol.* 1999;67:555–562.

18. Baker T. B,. Piper ME, McCarthy DE, Majeskie MR, Fiore MC. Addiction motivation reformulated: an affective processing model of negative reinforcement. *Psychol Rev.* 2004;111:33–51.

19. Waters AJ, Shiffman S, Sayette MA, Paty JA, Gwaltney C. G, Balabanis MH. Attentional bias predicts outcome in smoking cessation. *Health Psychol.* 2003;22:378–387.

20. Vidrine JI, Businelle MS, Cinciripini P, Li Y, Marcus MT, Waters AJ, Reitzel LR, Wetter DW. Associations of mindfulness with nicotine dependence, withdrawal, and agency. *Subs Abuse.* 2009;30:318–327.

21. Radloff L. The CES-D Scale: a self-report depression scale for research in the general population. *Appl Psychol Measure.* 1977;1:385–401.

22. Baer R, Smith G, Allen K. Assessment of mindfulness by self-report: The Kentucky Inventory of Mindfulness Skills. *Assessment.* 2004;11:191–206.

23. Wetter DW, Carmack CL, Anderson CB, Moore CA, De Moor CA, Cinciripini PM, Hirshkowitz M. Tobacco withdrawal signs and symptoms among women with and without a history of depression. *Exp Clin Psychopharmacol.* 2000;8: 88–96.

24. Watson D, Clark LA, Tellegen A. Development and validation of brief measures of positive and negative affect: The PANAS scale. *J Person Soc Psychol* 1988;54:1063–1070.

25. Cohen S, Kamarck T, Mermelstein R. A global measure of perceived stress. *J Health Soc Behav.* 1983;24: 385–396.

26. Wetter DW, Smith SS, Kenford SL, Jorenby DE, Fiore MC, Hurt RD, Offord KP, Barker TB. Smoking outcome expectancies: factor structure, predictive validity, and discriminant validity. *J Abnorm Psychol.* 1994;103:801–811.

27. Robinson TE, Berridge KC. The neural basis of craving: an incentive-sensitization theory of addiction. *Brain Res Rev.* 1993;18:247–291.

28. Wiers RW, Stacy AW, eds. *Handbook of Implicit Cognition and Addiction.* Thousand Oaks, CA: Sage Publications; 2006.

29. Cox WM, Fadardi JS, Pothos EM. The addiction-Stroop test: theoretical considerations and procedural recommendations. *Psychol Bull.* 2006;132:443–476.

30. Swanson JE, Rudman LA, Greenwald AG. Using the Implicit Association Test to investigate attitude-behaviour consistency for stigmatized behaviour. *Cogn Emot.* 2001;15:207–230.

31. Gemar MC, Segal ZV, Sagrati, S, Kennedy SJ. Mood-induced changes on the Implicit Association Test in recovered depressed patients. *J Abnorm Psychol.* 2001;110:282–289.

32. Williams JMG, Mathews A, MacLeod C. The emotional Stroop task and psychopathology. *Psychol Bull.* 1996;120:3–24.

33. Ostafin BD, Marlatt GA. Surfing the urge: experiential acceptance moderates the relation between automatic alcohol motivation and hazardous drinking. *J Soc Clin Psychol.* 2008;27:404–418.

34. Schneider W, Eschman A, Zuccolotto A. *E-Prime User's Guide.* Pittsburgh: Psychology Software Tools; 2002.

35. de Houwer J. The Implicit Association Test as a tool for studying dysfunctional associations in psychology. *Behav Ther Exp Psychol.* 2002;53:115–133.

36. Waters AJ, Carter BL, Robinson JD, Wetter DW, Lam CY, Cinciripini PM. Implicit attitudes to smoking are associated with craving and dependence. *Drug Alcohol Depend.* 2007;91:178–186.

37. Greenwald AG, Nosek A, Banaji MR. Understanding and using the Implicit Association Test: 1. An improved scoring algorithm. *J Person Soc Psychol.* 2003;85:197–216.

38. McKenna FP. Sharma D. Reversing the emotional Stroop effect: the role of fast and slow components. *J Exp Psychol Learn Memory Cogn.* 2004;30:382–392.

39. Waters AJ, Sayette MA, Franken IHA, Schwartz J. Generalizability of carry-over effects in the emotional Stroop task. *Behav Res Ther.* 2005;43:715–732.

40. Phaf RH, Kan K-J. The automaticity of emotional Stroop: a meta-analysis. *J Behav Ther Exp Psychiatry.* 2007;38:184–199.

41. Kucera H, Francis WN. *Computational Analysis of Present Day American English.* Providence, RI: Brown University Press; 1967.

42. Havlicek LL, Peterson NL. Effect of the violation of assumptions upon significance levels of the Pearson r. *Psychol Bull.* 1977;84:373–377.

43. Waters AJ, Sayette MA. Implicit cognition and tobacco addiction. In: RW. Wiers RW, Stacy AW, eds. *Handbook on Implicit Cognition and Addiction.* Thousand Oaks, CA: Sage; 2006:309–338.

INTRODUCTION

Mindfulness-Based Therapies for Substance Use Disorders: Part 2

This is the second of 2 Special Issues of *Substance Abuse* devoted to mindfulness meditation–based interventions for substance use disorders (SUDs) and their spectrum. The first part was published as the December 2009 issue of *Substance Abuse* (1). It featured 5 articles describing results of studies evaluating mindfulness-based interventions: a systematic review of literature on this topic, by Zgierska et al. (2), and 4 original research papers by Bowen et al. (3), Brewer et al. (4), Vidrine et al. (5) and Waters et al. (6). Combined, findings from these pilot-level studies suggest that mindfulness meditation–based interventions may be efficacious for SUDs.

This second Special Issue further adds to the mindfulness literature by presenting results of 5 additional studies that evaluated effects of mindfulness-based interventions in a range of substance-abusing client populations. Papers in this issue illustrate the ways in which mindfulness practice has been combined with other behavioral treatments and/or adapted to meet the needs of specific client populations.

In their study "Linguistic Analysis to Assess the Effect of a Mindfulness Intervention on Self-Change for Adults in Substance Use Recovery," Liehr and colleagues used an innovative method to measure self-change in participants in a therapeutic community who received Mindfulness-Based Therapeutic Community (MBTC) versus treatment as usual. They used a linguistic analysis method applied to participant-written stories

of stress and found that the MBTC group used fewer negative words than the control group over all time points.

Britton and colleagues, in the study "The Contribution of Mindfulness Practice to a Multicomponent Behavioral Sleep Intervention Following Substance Abuse Treatment in Adolescents: A Treatment-Development Study," found that mindfulness practice was associated with improved sleep, psychological health, and reduced substance use.

In "Psychosocial Treatment for Methamphetamine Use Disorders: A Preliminary Randomized Controlled Trial of Cognitive Behavior Therapy and Acceptance and Commitment Therapy," Smout and colleagues found that although Acceptance and Commitment Therapy (ACT) did not improve treatment outcomes or attendance compared to cognitive behavior therapy (CBT), it may be a viable therapeutic alternative for methamphetamine use disorders.

In their article "Development of an Acceptance-Based Coping Intervention for Alcohol Dependence Relapse Prevention," Vieten and colleagues describe the development and pilot testing of a mindfulness-based relapse prevention intervention for alcohol dependent individuals who stopped drinking within the past 6 months.

Amaro and colleagues, in their study "Addiction Treatment Intervention: An Uncontrolled Prospective Pilot Study of Spiritual Self-Schema Therapy with Latina Women," noted high rates of intervention acceptability, and positive changes in outcomes relevant to human immunodeficiency virus (HIV) prevention and recovery from addiction.

Although conclusive data for mindfulness meditation–based interventions as therapies for SUDs are lacking, the preliminary evidence reported in these and prior studies suggests their efficacy. The promise of mindfulness-based therapies is supported by the consistency of positive results demonstrated across different study designs, intervention modalities, subject populations, and addictive disorders treated (2). Additional support for the potential efficacy of these interventions in SUDs can be drawn from the results of studies of other clinical conditions: mindfulness-based therapies have been shown effective or potentially effective for a variety of medical and mental health disorders, including stress, anxiety, depression, emotion dysregulation, and avoidance coping (7–12), all known risk factors for relapse in SUDs (13, 14). In this context, mindfulness meditation–based interventions may be particularly helpful for patients with co-occurring substance use and mental health disorders ("dual diagnosis").

In addition, mindfulness-based interventions appear safe, satisfying to clients, and may have long-lasting effects in the context of continued meditation practice (2, 7)—all vital qualities of an "ideal" treatment. The success of mindfulness-based interventions and the unsatisfactory outcomes of many existing therapeutic modalities indicate that the time is right for rigorous assessment of mindfulness-based therapies for addictive disorders.

REFERENCES

1. Marcus M, Zgierska A. Mindfulness-based therapies for substance use disorders: part 1. *Subst Abus.* 2009;30:263–265.

2. Zgierska A, Rabago D, Chawla N, Kushner K, Koehler R, Marlatt A. Mindfulness meditation for substance use disorders: a systematic review. *Subst Abus.* 2009;30:266–294.

3. Bowen S, Chawla N, Collins SE, et al. Mindfulness-based relapse prevention for substance use disorders: a pilot efficacy trial. *Subst Abus.* 2009;30:295–305.

4. Brewer JA, Sinha R, Chen JA, et al. Mindfulness training and stress reactivity in substance abuse: results from a randomized, controlled stage I pilot study. *Subst Abus.* 2009;30:306–317.

5. Vidrine JI, Businelle MS, Cinciripini P, et al. Associations of mindfulness with nicotine dependence, withdrawal, and agency. *Subst Abus.* 2009;30:318–327.

6. Waters AJ, Reitzel LR, Cinciripini P, et al. Associations between mindfulness and implicit cognition and self-reported affect. *Subst Abus.* 2009;30:328–337.

7. Baer RA. Mindfulness training as a clinical intervention: a conceptual and empirical review. *Clin Psychol Sci Prac.* 2003;10:125–143.

8. Hayes SC, Luoma JB, Bond FW, Masuda A, Lillis J. Acceptance and commitment therapy: model, processes and outcomes. *Behav Res Ther.* 2006;44:1–25.

9. Davidson RJ, Kabat-Zinn J, Schumacher J, et al. Alterations in brain and immune function produced by mindfulness meditation. *Psychosom Med.* 2003;65:564–570.

10. Grossman P, Niemann L, Schmidt S, Walach H. Mindfulness-based stress reduction and health benefits. A meta-analysis. *J Psychosom Res.* 2004;57:35–43.

11. Praissman S. Mindfulness-based stress reduction: a literature review and clinician's guide. *J Am Acad Nurse Pract.* Apr;20:212–216.

12. Tang YY, Ma Y, Wang J, et al. Short-term meditation training improves attention and self-regulation. *Proc Natl Acad Sci U S A.* 2007;104:17152–17156.

13. Ciraulo DA, Piechniczek-Buczek J, Iscan EN. Outcome predictors in substance use disorders. *Psychiatr Clin North Am.* 2003;26:381–409.

14. Fox HC, Bergquist KL, Hong KI, Sinha R. Stress-induced and alcohol cue-induced craving in recently abstinent alcohol-dependent individuals. *Alcohol Clin Exp Res.* 2007;31:395–403.

Aleksandra Zgierska, MD, PhD
Department of Family Medicine
University of Wisconsin, School of Medicine
and Public Health, Madison, WI

Marianne T. Marcus, EdD, RN, FAAN
Center for Substance Abuse Education,
Prevention, and Research
University of Texas Health Science
Center-Houston School of Nursing
Houston, TX

Linguistic Analysis to Assess the Effect of a Mindfulness Intervention on Self-Change for Adults in Substance Use Recovery

Patricia Liehr, PhD, RN
Marianne T. Marcus, EdD, RN, FAAN
Deidra Carroll, BS
L. Kian Granmayeh, BA
Stanley G. Cron, MSPH
James W. Pennebaker, PhD

ABSTRACT. Substance use is a pervasive health problem. Therapeutic community (TC) is an established substance abuse treatment but TC environments are stressful and dropout rates are high. Mindfulness-based TC (MBTC) intervention was developed to address TC stress and support self-change that could impact treatment retention. Self-change was assessed through feeling and thinking word-use in written stories of stress from 140 TC residents in a historical control group and 253 TC residents in a MBTC intervention group. Data were collected 5 times over a 9-month period. Linguistic analysis showed no differences between the groups over time; however, over all time points, the MBTC intervention group used fewer negative emotion words than the TC control group. Also, negative emotion ($P < .01$) and anxiety ($P < .01$) word-use decreased whereas positive emotion word-use increased ($P < .05$) over time in both groups. Descriptive data from linguistic analyses indicated that sustained self-change demands participation in mindfulness behaviors beyond the instructor-guided MBTC intervention.

Patricia Liehr is affiliated with the Christine E. Lynn College of Nursing, Florida Atlantic University, Boca Raton, Florida, USA.

Marianne T. Marcus, Deidra Carroll, L. Kian Granmayeh, and Stanley G. Cron are affiliated with the Center of Substance Abuse Education, Prevention, and Research, The University of Texas Health Science Center–Houston, School of Nursing, Houston, Texas, USA.

James W. Pennebaker is affiliated with the Department of Psychology, University of Texas, Austin, Texas, USA.

This study was supported by National Institute on Drug Abuse grant DA R01 DA017719 to Dr. Marianne T. Marcus. The authors are grateful to the administration, staff, and clients of the Houston facility of Cenikor Foundation for their participation. They also thank the dedicated Mindfulness-Based Stress Reduction instructors, Michele Fine, Linda Safranek, Susan Wolfe, and Patricia Palmer, without whose commitment and assistance the study would not have been possible. The MBTC manual is available from Dr. Marianne Marcus at Marianne.T.Marcus@uth.tmc.edu

INTRODUCTION

Substance use is a pervasive health problem for the American population and worldwide. More than 20 million Americans abuse substances (1) and the cost to the nation extends beyond personal health, affecting families and communities. There are effective treatments for substance abuse, including pharmacologic and behavioral approaches (2). Therapeutic community (TC), a behavioral approach, has an established place in the repertoire of substance abuse treatment (3, 4). TC provides a highly structured social learning environment, where the community is the key agent for behavioral change. Studies have shown that people who complete TC treatment have lower levels of substance abuse, criminal behavior, unemployment, and depression than they had prior to treatment (5–8). However, dropout rates can be as high as 50% and dropout is most prevalent in the first 30 to 60 days of treatment (9). It is critical to improve treatment retention and to begin to understand self-change processes affecting it.

Stress is one factor that demands consideration when assessing dropout in TC settings. Although there are few data linking stress to the TC environment, studies of similar restrictive hierarchical settings, such as prisons (10) and military training camps (11), have identified chronic stress as an inherent dimension of these environments. With stress as a therapeutic goal, a mindfulness-based therapeutic community (MBTC) intervention was developed (12, 13), merging mindfulness-based stress reduction (MBSR) (14) and TC treatment (12) modalities. MBSR is commonly used for physical and mental health problems, including stress-related conditions (15). The TC and MBSR philosophies share common ground principles, such as a focus on the present moment, nonjudgmental acceptance, and attention to the whole person (12). For individuals who have continually tried to alter their circumstances with psychoactive substances, the present-centered, nonjudgmental way of being, endorsed by the MBTC intervention, can be a major whole-self shift that demands exploration. Within the context of TC treatment, the underlying assumption regarding the "whole person" nature of substance use dis-

orders suggests that self-change is necessary in areas of socialization, cognitive and emotional skills, and psychological development (16) if sustained recovery is to occur. TC treatment generally requires between 6 and 12 months of living in a residential community, where thoughts, feelings, and behaviors are regularly discussed. Whereas change in behavior is observable as it is enforced through the TC "rules and tools of right living," changes in thoughts and feelings are more elusive and seldom documented beyond anecdotal evidence. Formally collected stories may provide a perspective on thinking and feeling self-change. Stories are an integral dimension of many substance abuse treatments (17), and stories of stress are particularly relevant for people who are moving into the restrictive TC environment.

If change in thoughts and feelings could be documented through stories of stress, it may be possible to understand the self-change processes necessary for TC retention and, therefore, TC treatment success. In this instance, it may also be possible to evaluate the contribution of a MBSR-based program to the self-change experience of TC residents. Pennebaker and Stone have proposed word-use as empirical evidence of one's personality characteristics (18). They have developed a linguistic analysis method that can be readily applied in practice settings, enabling evaluation of "thinking" and "feeling" words (19), thereby providing perspective regarding self-change processes.

The purpose of this analysis was to explore effects of the newly developed MBTC intervention, a tailored therapy merging MBSR with TC treatment, on self-change processes ("thinking" and "feeling" word-use in written stories of stress) in the TC setting, over a 9-month study period.

METHODS

Design

This article reports findings of linguistic analysis applied to stress stories written by participants of a phase I behavioral therapies trial (12, 13). Primary focus of this trial was to evaluate whether the MBTC intervention was efficacious for reducing stress and improving retention among TC residents. The trial used a longitudinal historical control design. Data collection for the historical control phase of the trial was completed before the MBTC intervention phase was initiated. Standard-of-care TC treatment was delivered during the historical control phase of the study. In the MBTC intervention phase, a 6-week, instructor-guided mindfulness intervention was added to standard-of-care TC treatment (12, 13). Comparable data collection occurred during each phase of the trial. The historical control phase provided standard-of-care data for TC residents prior to implementation of the MBTC intervention. Therefore, each group, both the historical control and the MBTC intervention, had baseline data collected as well as 1-, 3-, 6-, and 9-month data. Self-change, measured through word-use in written stories of stress, was one of the outcome indicators for this trial.

Sample

All adults, 18 years and older, who entered a single TC facility in Southern United States were invited to participate in the study within the first 72 hours of their TC residency. The study was explained by one of the researchers (L.G. or D.C.) and informed consent was signed prior to data collection. Historical control subjects were enrolled from January 2005 through January 2006; intervention subjects were enrolled from February 2006 through November 2006. The study was approved by the University of Texas Health Science Center at Houston Institutional Review Board.

Outcome Measures: Stories of Stress as Indicators of Self-Change

At each data collection point (baseline, 1, 3, 6, and 9 months post entry), participants were asked to write a story about the stress they were experiencing. The writing instructions, following the Pennebaker et al.'s protocol (19), were:

> For the next 15 minutes write about thoughts and feelings regarding stressful issues in your life. Tell us about the issues; what do you think about them; what do you

feel about them; and, tell us how you are managing them. Don't worry about grammar or spelling or sentence structure. The most important thing is to let us know how things are going for you in relation to stress in your life. All your writing will be completely confidential. The only rule is that once you begin writing, continue to do so until your time is up. If you run out of things to write, just repeat what you've already written. It is important to keep writing for the entire time.

Preparing Stories of Stress for Analysis

The written stories of stress were transcribed and prepared for analysis using Linguistic Inquiry and Word Count (LIWC) software (19), a word-based computerized text analysis that discerns 72 linguistic categories. The validity of word categories has been extensively tested using panels of judges, factor analysis methods, and criterion-related validity procedures (20). The LIWC program reports word-use in percentages, indicating the number of words used in a particular category, relative to all the words used by a particular participant. In this analysis, the positive and negative emotion (feeling) and the cognitive process (thinking) word categories were included as outcome indicators. In addition, the anxiety word category and a combined inhibition and insight word category were used to better understand self-change processes related to stress. In previous research, the combined category of inhibition and insight had a positive correlation ($r = .71$) with recovery outcomes for a substance abuse population in a residential treatment facility (21). Table 1 provides examples of words in the LIWC dictionary associated with each selected word category; it also includes alpha reliabilities for each category estimated with 270 writings from a similar sample of participants (20).

Analysis

Descriptive statistics, including means, standard deviations, frequencies, and percentages were calculated for demographic and word-use variables at each time point. Repeated measures

TABLE 1. Selected Word Categories from the Linguistic Inquiry and Word Count (LIWC) Narrative Analysis Program with Associated Alpha Reliabilities and Example Words

Word category	Alpha	Example words
Positive emotion	.84	fun, grateful, vigor, love, secure, comfort
Negative emotion	.84	Whine, dislike, tense, neglect, worry, argue
● Anxiety	.77	Unsure, upset, restless, pressure, confused
Cognitive process	.84	Cause, discover, recognize, wonder, think
● Inhibition	.74	Control, forbid, hesitate, wait, stop
● Insight	.77	Accept, admit, analyze, examine, understand

analyses of change over time in word-use categories were conducted with linear mixed models (22) using SAS for Windows, version 9.1 (23). The level of significance for all statistical tests was set at 2-tailed $P < .05$. Values for positive emotion, negative emotion, and anxiety word-use did not follow a normal distribution, therefore, a square root transformation (24) was applied to adjust these variables prior to repeated measures analysis.

RESULTS

Figure 1 provides a flow chart indicating the participant numbers over the study course. The

FIGURE 1. Flowchart of participant numbers over time for the historical control therapeutic community (TC) group and the mindfulness-based therapeutic community (MBTC) group.

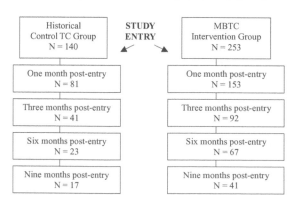

average age of participants at study entry was 35.1 (10.0) years. The majority was white (56%) and male (82%); 30% were black and 13% were Hispanic. Over the 9 months of the study, retention rates were 58%, 29%, 16%, and 12% for the TC control group, and 60%, 36%, 27%, and 16% for the MBTC intervention group at 1, 3, 6 and 9 months, respectively.

Thinking and feeling word-use was explored over a 9-month period (Table 2) as an indicator of personal change for adults receiving the TC control condition or the MBTC intervention. No statistically significant differences occurred between the groups over time in thinking and feeling word-use. Positive emotion word-use increased ($P < .05$), and negative emotion ($P < .01$) and anxiety ($P < .01$) word-use decreased over time regardless of group status. Overall, without consideration for time (e.g., average word-use across all data collection points), the MBTC intervention group used a smaller percentage of negative emotion words ($P < .05$) in stories of stress than the TC control group. There were no within- or between-group differences for thinking word-use, including the combined inhibition-insight word category.

DISCUSSION

The MBTC intervention did not significantly change feeling and thinking word-use over time; however, during the study period, the MBTC intervention group used altogether fewer negative emotion words when writing about stress compared to the TC control group. Over time, all participants, regardless of group status, used fewer negative emotion words and more positive emotion words when writing about stress.

The negative findings for differences between the TC control group and the MBTC intervention group over time can be viewed through at least 2 perspectives. The first suggests that the MBTC intervention was no more effective than TC alone in promoting self-change. Another perspective suggests that word-use in stories of stress was not sensitive to the MBTC intervention effect. If the first perspective is the chosen stance, concerns about the dwindling sample size and the possibility of a type II error surface. Perhaps if the entire

TABLE 2. Percentage of Feeling and Thinking Words Used Over Time

Word category	Baseline	1 month	3 months	6 months	9 months
Positive emotion*					
TC	2.1 (2.2)	2.6 (2.7)	2.4 (1.1)	2.1 (1.2)	2.4 (1.4)
MBTC	2.1 (1.6)	2.3 (1.6)	2.6 (1.7)	2.3 (1.3)	2.2 (1.3)
Negative emotion**					
TC	4.4 (3.0)	3.4 (2.1)	3.3 (1.8)	2.5 (1.5)	2.7 (1.4)
MBTC	4.0 (4.3)	3.3 (2.6)	2.5 (1.6)	2.4 (1.6)	2.5 (1.7)
Anxiety**					
TC	2.4 (2.8)	1.7 (1.9)	1.6 (1.4)	1.4 (1.5)	1.5 (1.5)
MBTC	2.0 (2.6)	1.8 (2.2)	1.2 (1.2)	1.2 (1.4)	1.3 (1.3)
Cognitive process (thinking)					
TC	7.9 (3.0)	8.5 (2.6)	8.3 (2.7)	8.2 (2.7)	8.7 (2.5)
MBTC	8.0 (3.0)	7.9 (2.3)	8.8 (2.8)	8.0 (2.4)	7.4 (2.4)
Inhibition and insight					
TC	2.9 (1.6)	3.1 (1.5)	3.0 (1.4)	2.5 (1.5)	3.2 (1.2)
MBTC	2.9 (1.6)	2.7 (1.4)	3.0 (1.6)	2.8 (1.5)	2.7 (1.6)

Note. Data are presented as mean (SD).
TC = standard of care therapeutic community; MBTC = mindfulness-based TC
*Significant change over 5 time points ($P < 0.05$); **significant change over 5 time points ($P < .01$), as evaluated using repeated measures analysis.

sample had been retained over time, differences would reach statistical significance. Descriptive statistics, summarizing word-use data, indicate that the greatest differences between the groups occurred at the 3-month measurement. These differences consistently favored the MBTC intervention group but differences disappeared by the 9-month measurement point.

Of note, the 3-month descriptive data collection time point coincided with a shift in the TC program activities when the scheduled instructor-guided mindfulness classes ended and the residents, regardless of group status, began employment outside the TC setting. This contextual information leads to questions about translating the instructor-guided MBTC intervention into everyday use. It is possible that the traditional TC environment, as it is currently configured, did not allow time or energy for formal and/or informal practice when participants resumed employment. Although guided meditation CDs were available, records indicated infrequent use by residents following the instructor-guided MBTC intervention. Like any behavioral therapy, participants must engage in the behavior if the effect is to be documented. Kabat-Zinn (15) addresses this point by noting that people do not have to like mindfulness practice, they "just have to do it" (p 41–42). At the

very least, these findings indicate a need for a better weaving of mindfulness practice into TC treatment throughout the resident's course of stay. The fact that the MBTC intervention group used fewer negative emotion words overall, whereas there were no significant group differences in word-use at baseline, may indicate that the MBTC participants differentially related to stress and negative emotions, suggesting that further study of the MBTC intervention is warranted.

The second perspective for considering insignificant differences between the groups is the possibility of lack of sufficient sensitivity of the word-use outcome measure. This explanation would be more plausible if it was inconsistent with other data measured at the same time points in this trial. However, the pattern of word-use change is consistent with the direction of change in other measures assessed in this study (13). For instance, self-reported stress level (reported elsewhere (13), measured by the Symptoms of Stress Inventory) decreased significantly over the study period regardless of group assignment, with the 3-month differences between the TC and the MBTC groups being most pronounced (13). Although it may be too early to dismiss linquistic analysis as an insensitive outcome indicator, our results do not provide strong support for its use in assessing the effect of the MBTC intervention.

The overall findings indicate significant changes in feeling word-use in both groups, unaccompanied by changes in thinking word use. In the current study, there was an a priori expectation that the MBTC intervention would facilitate more complex thinking, as reflected by increased thinking word-use, and improvement in positive and negative emotion word-use. Smyth and Pennebaker (25) report that expressive writing enables identification and labeling of feelings, a simple action that often results in a more "complex cognitive representation" (p. 3) of a circumstance. This composite of feeling and thinking self-change has been shown to correlate with improved health outcomes (25). Although negative emotion word-use decreased and positive emotion word-use increased in both groups over time, these changes in feeling word-use did not translate into significant changes in thinking word-use. The absence of thinking self-change leads to questions about "reperceiving," a cognitive capacity identified as central to mindfulness and essential to self-management activities (26).

> By developing the capacity to stand back and witness emotional states such as anxiety, we increase our 'degrees of freedom' in response to such states, effectively freeing ourselves from automatic behavioral patterns. Through reperceiving, we are no longer controlled by states such as anxiety or fear but are instead able to use them as information. We are able to attend to the emotion, and choose to self-regulate in ways that foster greater health and well being. (26, p. 380)

Reperceiving is a complex cognitive process that is considered developmental in nature. It is a "rotation in consciousness" (26) where subjective becomes objective. Reperceiving may not yet have become a habit for the MBTC intervention group by the 3-month time point, making it unlikely that the feeling word-use changes could be expressed as a measurable change in thinking word-use.

In conclusion, in this study, linguistic analysis of stress stories, written by the TC residents over the 9-month study period, did not reveal significant differences between the historical control group and experimental group that received the MBTC intervention. However, consideration of 3-month differences suggests that mindfulness must be practiced if its effect is to be noted. Care providers are challenged to identify manageable approaches to help TC residents sustain the practice of mindfulness. When this challenge is addressed, a more meaningful evaluation of the MBTC intervention, as a vehicle for creating self-change for adults in substance use recovery, can be pursued.

REFERENCES

1. SAMSHA. State estimates of substance use and mental health from the 2005–2006 National Surveys on Drug Use and Health. Table 1. Illicit drug use in past month, by age group and state. 2007. Available at: http://www.oas.samhsa.gov/2k6state/ageTabs.htm/. Accessed April 10, 2009.

2. Snow D, Delaney KR. Substance use and recovery: charting a course toward optimism. *Arc Psychiatr Nurs.* 2006;20:288–290.

3. Broekaert E. What future for the therapeutic community in the field of addiction? A view from Europe. *Addiction.* 2006;101:1677–1678.

4. Smith LA, Gates S, Foxcroft D. Therapeutic communities for substance related disorder. *Cochrane Database Syst Rev.* 2006;(1):CD005338.

5. Simpson DD, Joe DW, Brown BS. Treatment retention and follow up outcome in the Drug Abuse Treatment Outcome Study (DATOS). *Psychol Addict Behav.* 1997;11:294–307.

6. Simpson DD, Joe GW, Fletcher BW, Hubbard, RL, Anglin MD. A national evaluation of treatment outcomes for cocaine dependence. *Arch Gen Psychiatry.* 1999;56:507–514.

7. Martin SS, Butzin CA, Saum CA, Inciardi JA. Three year outcomes of the therapeutic community treatment for drug involved offenders in Delaware: from prison to work release to aftercare. *Prison J.* 1999;79:294–320.

8. Wexler HK, Melnick G, Lower L, Peters J. Three-year aftercare in California. *Prison J.* 1999;79:321–336.

9. DeLeon G, Hawke J, Jainchill N, Melnick, G. Therapeutic communities: enhancing retention in treatment using "Senior Professor" staff. *J Subst Abuse Treat.* 2000;19:375–382.

10. Nurse J, Woodcock P, Ormsby J. Influence of environmental factors on mental health within prisons: focus group study. *BMJ.* 2003;327:480–484.

11. Lieberman HR, Tharion WJ, Shukitt-Hale B, Speckman KL, Tulley, R. Effects of caffeine, sleep loss, and stress

on cognitive performance and mood during US Navy SEAL training. *Psychopharmacology.* 2002;164:250–261.

12. Marcus MT, Liehr PR, Schmitz J, et al. Behavioral therapies trials: a case example. *Nurs Res.* 2007;56:210–216.

13. Marcus MT, Schmitz J, Moeller FG, et al. Mindfulness-based stress reduction in therapeutic community treatment: a stage 1 trial. *Am J Drug Alcohol Abuse.* 2009;35:103–108.

14. Kabat-Zinn J. *Wherever You Go There You Are.* New York: Hyperion; 1994.

15. Kabat-Zinn J. *Full Catastrophe Living.* New York: Dell; 1990.

16. DeLeon G. *The Therapeutic Community: Theory, Model, and Method.* New York: Springer; 2000.

17. Diamond J. *Narrative Means to Sober Ends.* New York: Guilford Press; 2002.

18. Pennebaker JW, Stone LD. Words of wisdom: language use over the life span. *J Pers Soc Psychol.* 2003;85:291–301.

19. Pennebaker JW, Francis ME, Booth RJ. *Linguistic Inquiry and Word Count (LIWC).* Mahwah, NJ: Erlbaum; 2001.

20. Pennebaker JW, King LA. Linguistic styles: language use as an individual difference. *J Pers Soc Psychol.* 1999;77:1296–1312.

21. Stephenson GM, Laszlo J, Ehmann B, Lefever RMH, Lefever R. Diaries of significant events: sociolinguistic correlates of therapeutic outcomes in patients with addiction problems. *J Community Appl Soc Psychol,* 1997;7:389–411.

22. Brown H, Prescott R. *Applied Mixed Models in Medicine.* 2nd ed. Hoboken, NJ: John Wiley & Sons; 2006.

23. Walker GA. *Common Statistical Methods for Clinical Research with SAS Examples.* 2nd ed. Cary, NC: SAS Institute; 2002.

24. Kirkwood BR, Sterne JAC. *Essential Medical Statistics.* 2nd ed. Malden, MA: Blackwell Science; 2003.

25. Smyth JM, Pennebaker JW. Exploring the boundary conditions of expressive writing: in search of the right recipe. *Br J Health Psychol,* 2008;13:1–7.

26. Shapiro SL, Carlson EE, Astin JA, Freedman B. Mechanisms of mindfulness. *J Clin Psychol,* 2006;62:373–386.

The Contribution of Mindfulness Practice to a Multicomponent Behavioral Sleep Intervention Following Substance Abuse Treatment in Adolescents: A Treatment-Development Study

Willoughby B. Britton, PhD
Richard R. Bootzin, PhD
Jennifer C. Cousins, PhD
Brant P. Hasler, MA
Tucker Peck, BS
Shauna L. Shapiro, PhD

ABSTRACT. Poor sleep is common in substance use disorders (SUDs) and is a risk factor for relapse. Within the context of a multicomponent, mindfulness-based sleep intervention that included mindfulness meditation (MM) for adolescent outpatients with SUDs ($n = 55$), this analysis assessed the contributions of MM practice intensity to gains in sleep quality and self-efficacy related to SUDs. Eighteen adolescents completed a 6-session study intervention and questionnaires on psychological distress, sleep quality, mindfulness practice, and substance use at baseline, 8, 20, and 60 weeks postentry. Program participation was associated with improvements in sleep and emotional distress, and reduced substance use. MM practice frequency correlated with increased sleep duration and improvement in self-efficacy about substance use. Increased sleep duration was associated with improvements in psychological distress, relapse resistance, and substance use–related problems. These findings suggest

Willoughby B. Britton is affiliated with the Department of Psychiatry and Human Behavior, Brown University Medical School, Providence, Rhode Island, USA.

Richard R. Bootzin and Tucker Peck are affiliated with the Department of Psychology, University of Arizona, Tucson, Arizona, USA.

Jennifer C. Cousins and Brant P. Hasler are affiliated with the Western Psychiatric Institute and Clinic of the University of Pittsburgh, Pittsburgh, Pennsylvania, USA.

Shauna L. Shapiro is affiliated with the Department of Counseling Psychology, Santa Clara University, Santa Clara, California, USA.

The authors would like to gratefully acknowledge the contributions of John Leggio, Patrick Borasso, Robert Miller, and Lucy Ledi for help in recruiting adolescents from their substance abuse treatment programs and the collaborative contributions of the research team members, Sally Stevens, Elaine Bailey, Sabrina Hitt, Michael Cameron, and Keith Fridel.

This study was supported by contract from the Office of the National Drug Control Policy (ONDCP). The views expressed in this article are those of the authors and do not necessarily reflect those of the funding agency.

that sleep is an important therapeutic target in substance abusing adolescents and that MM may be a useful component to promote improved sleep.

INTRODUCTION

There is robust evidence of a bidirectional relationship between substance abuse and sleep. Many substances of abuse produce disrupted sleep and daytime sleepiness, which in turn can promote further substance use to counter these effects (1). Emotional distress and poor sleep also have bidirectional causal pathways. Adolescents with psychological distress are more likely to develop sleep problems (2), and sleep problems in adolescents increase the risk for anxiety disorders, depression, and lower self-esteem (3–7).

Because of the interrelationship between poor sleep, emotional problems, and substance use, research has begun to explore whether cognitive-behavioral treatment of sleep disorders may be useful in the amelioration of emotional disturbances (8) or, conversely, if behavioral and pharmacological treatments for emotional disturbances may improve sleep (9). Because many adolescents who abuse substances are also anxious and depressed (10), targeting sleep disturbance for treatment has the potential benefit of improving treatment outcomes for both substance abuse and emotional functioning.

Mindfulness is a form of nonjudgmental present-moment awareness that can be cultivated through the practice of mindfulness meditation (MM). Mindfulness meditation is particularly relevant to sleep-related disorders because it serves the dual functions of reducing hyperarousal (11–13) and decreasing negative emotional states such as anxiety, depression, worry, and rumination (14–18) that are commonly reported problems among insomniacs (19). Preliminary studies have suggested that MM is associated with improvements in self-reported sleep disturbance (20–29), possibly by reducing stress and negative affect-related arousal, although the mechanism has remained unclear.

Mindfulness-based approaches are now being applied to substance abuse and addiction (30–34). With the recognition that stress, negative affect, and low distress tolerance are important triggers for relapse, mindfulness has been described as a process of desensitization to negative affect and as an exposure strategy that helps to extinguish automatic avoidance of negative emotions (i.e., substance use). "Repeated experience of observing rather than reacting to one's urges or emotional responses to eliciting stimuli may engender a greater sense of control over the actual decision to use" (35, p. 288).

With the rationale that improving sleep and daytime sleepiness could improve emotional functioning and reduce subsequent drug use, we developed a 6-session multicomponent sleep intervention to address sleep problems in adolescents who had recently completed substance abuse treatment and had residual sleep complaints (8). This intervention was a novel combination of 2 treatment packages: cognitive-behavioral therapy for insomnia, similar to the one described by Perlis et al. (36), and Mindfulness-Based Stress Reduction (MBSR) that features training in mindfulness meditation with a focus on stress reduction (37).

In the current paper, we report results from a prospective open clinical trial ($n = 55$) evaluating the overall effects of a multicomponent behavioral sleep intervention on self-reported sleep and daytime sleepiness, emotional distress, relapse resistance, and substance use and related harms at baseline, 8, 20, and 60 weeks postentry. In a secondary analysis of study completers who provided mindfulness practice data ($n = 18$), we evaluated MM practice patterns and their relationship to the primary outcome variables. Based on the existing literature, we hypothesized that MM practice will be associated with improved sleep/sleepiness, decreased emotional distress, increased relapse resistance, and decreased substance abuse.

METHODS

Design and Procedures

The study was a 60-week uncontrolled prospective clinical trial evaluating effects of a multicomponent behavioral sleep intervention. Following informed consent procedures and baseline assessments, participants entered a 6-session intervention, followed by posttreatment, 3- and 12-month follow-up assessments (at 8, 20, and 60 weeks postentry, respectively). The study was approved by the Institutional Review Board at the University of Arizona. Certificate of Confidentiality was provided by the National Institute of Drug Abuse.

In this article, the analyses appear in 2 parts. The main analysis briefly reports the study intervention effects on sleep, distress, and substance use in adolescents recently treated for substance abuse ($n = 55$). The secondary analysis aims to determine the contribution of mindfulness meditation practice amount to outcome variables in a subgroup of study completers ($n = 18$).

Participants

Eligibility criteria included adolescents ages 13 to 19 with complaints of current sleep problems or daytime sleepiness who completed an outpatient substance abuse treatment within the year before entering the study. Participants were recruited through 4 substance abuse treatment programs in Tucson, Arizona. These programs varied in treatment length and model. The study was described in written materials and over the telephone to parents who requested more information. Fifty-five eligible adolescents and their parents expressed interest in enrolling and were scheduled for an in-person meeting during which informed consent and baseline assessment were completed. Of the enrolled 55 subjects, 23 (42%) attended at least 4 of the 6 treatment sessions and were considered treatment completers. Secondary analysis included only treatment completers who both attended the last treatment

session and provided MM practice information ($n = 18$).

The Multicomponent Behavioral Sleep Intervention

We developed a manualized treatment for adolescents to improve sleep/sleepiness and emotional distress (38). The treatment consisted of 6 90-minute weekly small group sessions (2 to 6 subjects per group), with the first session dedicated to sleep education, and sessions 2 to 6 split equally between cognitive-behavioral and modified Mindfulness-Based Stress Reduction (MBSR) therapies. The cognitive-behavioral sleep treatment component consisted of stimulus control instructions, regularization of sleep-wake schedules, including the use of bright light therapy, and cognitive therapy. See Bootzin and Stevens (19) for detailed descriptions of each component.

The 5 mindfulness training sessions were derived from Mindfulness-Based Stress Reduction (MBSR) (37) but included some important modifications. Formal mindfulness practice homework consisted of 10 minutes/day, 6 days a week, of either sitting meditation or body scan meditation, but not mindful movement/yoga. Importantly, the explicit therapeutic goals of the program were stress reduction and sleep improvement and not substance abuse or relapse prevention, and the program did not include explicit addiction-related practices such as "urge surfing" or imagined cue exposure (39).

The intervention was manualized and the intervention session always had 2 Masters-level clinicians present, both of whom were trained by one of the authors (R.R.B.) in cognitive-behavioral component, and one of whom (in each treatment group) had received advanced training and had more than 1 year of experience in MBSR teaching. All sessions were taped and supervised by one of the authors (R.R.B.).

Measures

Participants completed all described outcome measures at baseline, 8, 20, and 60 weeks postentry. Emotional distress, relapse resistance, and substance use over the past 30 days were assessed using the Global Appraisal of Individual

Needs (GAIN) interview (40). The GAIN is a structured clinical interview, well-validated in adolescent substance-abusing populations (41, 42). The following 3 GAIN subscales were used:

1. The GAIN General Mental Distress Index (GMDI) is a 21-item scale that measures severity of depression, anxiety, somatic, and behavioral problems ($\alpha = .95$). Subscale scores range from 0 to 21, with scores ≥ 7 indicating a clinical level of medical or mental health problems.
2. The GAIN Self-Efficacy Index (SEI) is a 5-item scale that measures perceived likelihood of resisting substance use relapse. Scores range from 0 to 5, with higher scores indicating higher level of confidence about and motivation toward resisting relapse in different situations, and lower scores suggesting the need for assistance in daily living and/or a controlled environment. Confidence in dealing with high-risk situations has been found to predict posttreatment outcomes and likelihood of relapse (43).
3. The GAIN Substance Problem Index (SPI) is a 16-item measure that assesses severity of various symptoms associated with substance use, such as substance-related health and social problems ($\alpha = .88$). Its scores range from 0 to 16, with scores ≥ 4 indicating substance abuse, and ≥ 7 indicating dependence.

Frequency of drug use across 12 substance categories was assessed using the Drug Matrix Substance Frequency (SF), a subscale of the well-validated Risk Behavior Assessment questionnaire (44, 45). The SF scores range from 1 to 30, reflecting number of days of substance use within the last 30 days.

Severity of worry was assessed using the 16-item Penn State Worry Questionnaire (PSWQ) (46). The PSWQ shows sound psychometric properties in adolescents and young adults (47, 48). Its scores range from 16 to 80, with scores >45 indicating clinically significant levels of worry (49).

Self-reported daily sleep patterns were evaluated using the Sleep Diary. Estimates of sleep parameters from sleep diaries have been found to be reliable and valid in adults with insomnia (50). Collected measures included time in bed (TIB), sleep onset latency (SL), wake after sleep onset (WASO), and total sleep time (TST). In the current analyses, SL and WASO were combined into one measure of total wake time (TWT). Sleep efficiency (SE) represents the TST/TIB ratio (%), with <90% indicating poor sleep. The participants telephoned their daily sleep diaries into a voice-mail system and handed in hardcopies of the diaries weekly during the treatment period. Weekly averages at baseline and posttreatment were used in the analyses with a minimum of 3 days/week of valid data for inclusion. Significant improvements in completers in sleep diary variables, i.e., SL, TST, number of awakenings, WASO, sleep efficiency, and subjective sleep quality (all $P < .05$) from baseline to posttreatment have been previously reported (19, 51).

Severity of daytime sleepiness symptoms was assessed using the Epworth Sleepiness Scale (ESS) (52), an 8-item questionnaire in which participants rate the likelihood of dozing in different situations. The ESS has sound psychometric properties in adolescents ($\alpha = .88$) (53). Its scores range from 0 to 24, with a threshold ≥ 11 indicating pathological sleepiness.

MM practice frequency (number of practice sessions per week) and duration (minutes per practice session) were assessed at the final intervention session when participants were asked to estimate their average out-of-class MM practice.

Data Analysis

For the primary analysis ($n = 55$), separate repeated measures analysis of variance (ANOVAs) were used to assess the change in outcome variables across time, and the completer-noncompleter $\times$ treatment interaction. All variables were normally distributed. GAIN and questionnaire variables derived from SF, SPI, SEI, GMDI, worry, and ESS were 4-level within-subject variables (baseline, 8, 20, and 60 weeks). Between-subject variables were treatment completion status (completers ≥ 4 sessions) and gender (a higher percentage of girls completed treatment than boys).

The secondary analysis included completers who provided mindfulness practice data

($n = 18$). All variables within this subsample were normally distributed with the exception of SF and SPI that were skewed on some but not all time points (and therefore not transformed). Preliminary analyses examined baseline characteristics and possible differences between subgroups. The relationships between meditation amount (frequency and duration) and outcome variables were assessed with Spearman rank-order correlations, and by comparing outcome variables of completers who meditated (>once/week, $n = 10$) with completers who did not meditate (<once/week, $n = 8$) with repeated measures ANOVAs. Diary sleep outcome variables, derived from TST, TIB, SE, and TWT, were 2-level within-subject variables (pre, post). Multiple linear regression modeling was used to control for baseline differences and intervention session attendance. Spearman correlations were used to assess the predicted relationship between improvements in sleep, distress, and substance abuse. Statistical significance was set at alpha levels <.05 (2-tailed), although trends <.1 were reported due to the preliminary nature of the data and the goal to reduce type II error. Data was analyzed using SPSS 14.0 software. Results are reported as mean ± SD or number/percentage unless otherwise indicated.

RESULTS

Of the 55 adolescents who completed baseline assessments, 23 completed at least 4 of the 6 sessions and were considered completers. GAIN and questionnaire data for 8-, 20-, and 60-week assessments were collected from 49, 43, and 51 participants, respectively. Sleep diary data were available only from completers ($n = 23$). Eighteen completers attended the last intervention session and provided mindfulness practice data for the secondary analysis. Follow-up data from this subgroup were available from 18, 17, and 16 participants at each follow-up time point, respectively, with complete sleep diary data available from 15 of these subjects.

Detailed demographic and baseline data of the larger sample ($n = 55$) have been described and reported previously (19, 51). Completers ($n = 23$; 13 male, age 16.4 ± 1.2) had fewer TST minutes than noncompleters at baseline, but otherwise did not differ on any baseline variables.

Table 1 shows baseline characteristics for both meditating and nonmeditating completers included in the secondary analysis ($n = 18$). Meditators ($n = 10$) and nonmeditators ($n = 8$) did not differ on any measure. Scores in both groups indicated high levels of sleep disturbance and mental distress, and low levels of substance

TABLE 1. Baseline Characteristics of Secondary Analysis Sample ($N = 18$)

Measure	Sample ($N = 18$)	Meditators ($N = 10$)	Nonmeditators ($N = 8$)
Male, n (%)	9 (50%)	5 (50%)	4 (50%)
Age, years, mean (SD)	16.4 (1.3)	16.2 (0.9)	16.8 (1.5)
Sessions, n (SD)	5.1 (0.7)	5.2 (0.7)	5.0 (0.7)
TIB, minutes, mean (SD)	519.5 (83.7)	512.8 (74.9)	527.9 (98.1)
TST, minutes, mean (SD)	435.9 (65.3)	444.5 (61.8)	425.1 (72.2)
SE, percent, mean (SD)	0.85 (0.08)	0.87 (0.05)	0.81 (0.10)
GMDI, score, mean (SD)	10.9 (4.9)	10.4 (5.9)	11.6 (3.9)
SPI, score, mean (SD)	2.9 (4.1)	3.7 (4.8)	2.4 (3.7)
SF, score, mean (SD)	11.3 (17.8)	16.8 (22.3)	7.0 (11.8)
SEI, score, mean (SD)	3.2 (1.5)	3.5 (1.5)	2.9 (1.6)
Worry, score, mean (SD)	35.9 (10.2)	34.2 (11.2)	38.0 (9.2)
ESS, score, mean (SD)	8.2 (4.5)	8.6 (5.1)	7.8 (4.0)

Note. Meditator = 1+ practice session/week); nonmeditator =<1 practice session/week.
Sessions = number of treatment sessions attended; TIB = time in bed (minutes); TST = total sleep time (minutes); SE = sleep efficiency (%); GMDI = General Mental Distress Index; SPI = Substance Problem Index; SF = Substance Frequency (days used in last month); SEI = Self-Efficacy Index; Worry = Penn State Worry Questionnaire: ESS = Epworth Sleepiness Scale.
Meditators and nonmeditators did not differ on any measure at baseline.

FIGURE 1. Substance Frequency (SF) of the whole sample during the study period—frequency of substance use in the last 30 days. Females: $n = 16$; completers 10, noncompleters 6. Completer-noncompleter × time interaction: $F(3, 42) = 4.29$, $P = .01$. Males: $n = 24$; completers 10, noncompleters 14. Time main effect: $F(3, 66) = 11.3$, $P < .001$.*$P < .05$.

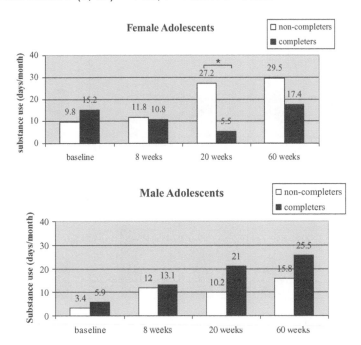

use–related problems, daytime sleepiness and worry at baseline.

Main Outcomes: Sleep, Substance Abuse, and Emotional Distress

Substance use frequency increased for all participants ($n = 55$) over all follow-up time points ($F(3, 34) = 7.8$, $P = .0004$), with a significant time × completer × sex interaction ($F(3, 34) = 4.6$, $P = .01$). Severity of substance use–related problems did not change significantly with time or completer status, but was also suggestive of gender-related interactions ($F(3, 35) = 2.4$, $P = .08$).

Figures 1 and 2 show substance use frequency and severity of substance use–related problems, assessed for the prior 30 days and during the study, separately for males and females, completers and noncompleters. Female adolescent completers reduced their substance use and substance-related problems through the 20-week follow-up but increased at 60 weeks ($F(3, 42) = 4.3$, $P = .01$), whereas the male teens and female noncompleters increased substance use at each time point ($F(3, 66) = 11.3$, $P < .001$). Regarding SPI-assessed severity of substance use–related problems, males peaked at 20 weeks, but then reported fewer problems at 60 weeks, although their overall level of substance use was high (time main effect, $F(3, 69) = 3.0$, $P < .05$).

With regard to emotional distress, GMDI scores improved significantly for all participants and improvements were sustained across all follow-up time points ($F(3, 37) = 13.3$, $P < .001$). Completers showed a trend to improve their GMDI scores more than noncompleters ($F(1, 47) = 2.9$, $P = .09$) from pre- to post-treatment. Sleepiness severity decreased more in completers than noncompleters over all follow-up time points ($F(3, 34) = 2.9$, $P = .05$), but did not decrease for all participants as a whole ($F(3, 34) = 2.2$, $P = .11$).

FIGURE 2. Substance Problem Index (SPI) of the whole sample during the study period. Females: $n = 16$; completers 10, noncompleters 6. No significant effects. Males: $n = 25$, completers 10, noncompleters 15. Time main effect: $F(3, 69) = 3.0$, $P < .05$.

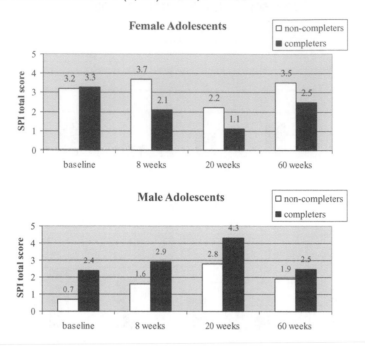

Secondary Analysis (n = 18): Mindfulness Meditation Practice and Its Relationship to Primary Outcomes

MM practice pattern. In addition to 30 minutes of in-class practice time, participants were asked to complete a MM homework consisting of MM practice for 10 minutes once a day, 6 days/week, for a total recommended "dose" of 60 minutes per week outside of class. Adolescents in this study reported practicing approximately 25% to 30% of the recommended time (15 to 20 minutes/week). On average, they practiced 5 to 10 minutes/day, 1 to 2 days/week, for a total of approximately 15 to 20 minutes/week outside of class (16.8 ± 5.0 minutes). However, there was great variability in outside MM practice. Eight (44%) subjects reported practicing less than once a week or not at all. Out of the 10 who reported meditating more than once a week, 28% reported meditating 1 to 2 times, and 28% reported meditating ≥ 3 times a week. For the majority of those who meditated outside of class (68%), meditation practice duration was typically less than 15 minutes; only 3 (17%) reported meditating for 15 to 30 minutes each time.

Relationship Between MM Practice and Outcomes

In line with predictions, frequency of practice was strongly and positively correlated with TIB, TST, and self-efficacy scores ($P < .05$), and negatively, but nonsignificantly correlated with distress, worry, drug use, and substance-related problem scores at posttreatment. Practice duration was not correlated with any outcome variable at any time point.

Meditation practice frequency was associated with increases in reported TST ($r = .56$, $P = .02$) and TIB ($r = .66$, $P = .01$) from baseline to postintervention (8 weeks postentry). Over the course of the 6-session intervention, TST increased by a mean of 74 ± 88.6 minutes in those who meditated regularly (more than once a week, $n = 9$), and decreased by a mean of 27 ± 103.3 minutes in those who meditated less than once a week ($n = 6$; $F(1, 13) = 5.7$, $P = .03$) (see Figure 3).

FIGURE 3. Total sleep time (mean minutes ± SD) at baseline and 8 weeks postentry in meditating ($n = 9$) and nonmeditating ($n = 6$) completers. Meditator = 1+ practice session/week, nonmeditator =<1 practice session/week. Meditator-nonmeditator × time interaction: $F(1, 13) = 5.7$, $P = .03$. *$P < .05$.

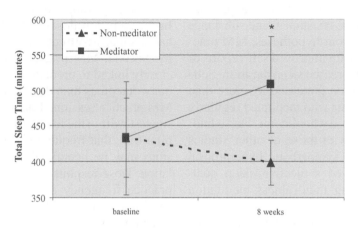

Frequency of MM practice during the intervention was associated with higher self-efficacy scores at 20 ($r = .50$, $P = .02$) and 60 ($r = .60$, $P = .01$) weeks. Compared to nonmeditators, adolescents who practiced MM regularly ($n = 10$) had higher self-efficacy scores at 20 weeks ($t(15)=2.5$, $P = .03$); these differences were not significant at 60 weeks ($t(15) = 1.7$, $P = .10$).

MM Practice and Sleep: Covariates

In addition to MM practice intensity, other variables (e.g., baseline sleep duration) and concomitant cognitive-behavioral sleep therapy could have influenced treatment outcomes. To test this possibility, change in TST was entered into a regression analysis as the dependent variable, with meditation frequency, baseline TST, and number of intervention sessions attended as independent variables. Frequency of meditation practice significantly predicted a longer posttreatment TST even after these variables were controlled for ($P = .01$). Number of treatment sessions attended (which indicated number of cognitive-behavioral intervention sessions) did not predict changes in any sleep variable.

Relationships Between Sleep, Emotional Functioning, and Substance Use

Based on our study rationale that improving sleep could improve emotional functioning and reduce subsequent substance use, we investigated the relationship between improvements in sleep, distress, relapse resistance, and substance use in the secondary analysis subsample ($n = 18$). In line with predictions, increases in TST were correlated with decreases in worry at posttreatment ($r = -.49$, $P = .05$), and higher self-efficacy ($r = .70$, $P = .005$) and decreased substance use–related problems at 20 weeks ($r = -.56$, $P = .02$).

No side effects or adverse events were reported during the study.

DISCUSSION

Results of this open, prospective, treatment-development trial, presented in the current and previous analyses (19, 51, 54), suggest that a multicomponent intervention, including both cognitive-behavioral therapy and MM training, can improve sleep, emotional distress, and substance use–related outcomes in adolescent substance abuse outpatients, and that MM practice intensity may be a significant factor contributing to these improvements.

The current analyses focused on the contribution of MM practice (frequency and duration) on the outcome variables of sleep, emotional distress, relapse resistance, and substance use. Consistent with our hypotheses, MM practice was associated with improved self-reports of sleep, particularly increased sleep duration. Self-reported sleep duration increased by more than an hour for adolescents who meditated regularly and decreased for those who did not. These findings are consistent with those of other studies indicating decreased sympathetic hyperarousal (14–18) and improved subjective sleep quality (20–29) following mindfulness meditation training.

Although participants showed an overall sustained improvement in emotional distress, MM practice intensity was not strongly associated with these changes. One explanation is that MM is not intended to reduce negative emotions, only to improve acceptance of them so they do not unconsciously dictate automatic avoidance reactions (i.e., use of substances to change unwanted mental states). In line with this idea, MM practice was strongly predictive of self-efficacy and relapse resistance. This supports previous theories from mindfulness-based addiction literature that MM-related enhancements in self-awareness and distress tolerance may promote relapse resistance (35).

In our study, improvements in sleep were associated with improvements in psychological distress, self-efficacy, and substance use–related problems. Two previous analyses from the same study found that improvements in sleep were associated with decrease in traumatic stress symptoms (54) and better emotion regulation ability, specifically in regard to aggressive thoughts and actions, including suicidal ideation (51). Together with the current findings, they suggest that sleep quality may be an important factor in mindfulness meditation–related improvements in attention, emotional disturbance, and affect regulation (55–58).

The issue of meditation "dosage" warrants a special mention. First, the amount of meditation practice noted in this study (5 to 10 minutes/day, 1 to 2 times/week) is relatively low compared to other studies that implemented MBSR or Mindfulness-Based Cognitive Therapy (MBCT) interventions. Yet, the present data suggest that even such low "doses" can have some effects, even on physiological processes such as sleep. In our study, low doses of MM practice may have had a soporific effect on subjective sleep quality. Second, MM practice frequency was more closely linked to predicted improvements in primary outcomes than duration of each individual MM practice session. Taken together, these data suggest, within the limitations of an uncontrolled pilot trial, that frequent short MM practice sessions may be beneficial, at least in this population. Dose-response–related issues, both MM practice frequency and duration and practice-specific effects, should be considered in future research.

The method of extracting one component of a multicomponent intervention also deserves consideration. Using correlations between meditation practice intensity and outcome variables is a common approach in meditation research (59–65), and has been used to assess the relationships between practice amount and changes in sleep (24, 27), even within the context of a multicomponent behavioral sleep program (66, 67). This system of practice-outcome correlation is imperfect because meditation practice amount may be correlated with other variables such as personality characteristics or situational circumstances, e.g., overall treatment compliance or other behavioral changes. Because differences in meditation practice are self-selected, the causal direction could be reversed; i.e., those who most improve their sleep may become "better" meditators due to improved emotional and cognitive resources.

It should be noted that MBSR and MBCT (as well as programs that include them) are multicomponent cognitive-behavioral interventions and include social support and assertiveness/communication training, automatic thought, emotion and stress reactivity records, and yoga (exercise). In these interventions, meditation practice reflects only one component that may or may not be correlated with subject engagement in other components. Future research in which intensity of meditation is experimentally varied and individual intervention components are experimentally dismantled is needed to address these issues.

Study limitations included lack of a control group, small sample size, limited power, and high attrition. The study would have also benefited from more precise, daily, and nonretrospective meditation practice logs that delineated not only quantity but also type of practice, and were independent of possible social desirability biases. The addition of a measure evaluating degree of mindfulness, assessment of compliance with sleep-related homework assignments, and sleep and mindfulness practice during the follow-up period would also strengthen the design. In this study, the multicomponent intervention was provided after the substance abuse treatment had been completed; gains attributed to the study intervention could have also resulted from this prior substance abuse treatment or could represent natural disease course. Separating the substance abuse and sleep treatments also caused a number of practical problems, such as the ending of judicial oversight of the teens, making early attrition more likely. In future studies, it may be desirable to combine the multicomponent intervention with concomitant substance abuse treatment to maximize gains and possibly to reduce attrition.

In summary, participation in the mindfulness-based multicomponent behavioral sleep treatment was associated with improvements in sleep, emotional distress severity, and substance use recidivism rate. Study results suggest that a low dose of mindfulness meditation practice could have contributed to increases in sleep duration and improvement in self-efficacy about substance abuse. Increased sleep duration was associated with improvements in distress, relapse resistance, and substance-related problems. These findings, together with prior analyses from this study, suggest that sleep is an important therapeutic target for reducing substance abuse and that MM may be a useful therapy to promote improved sleep.

REFERENCES

1. Gillin J, Drummond S, Clark C, Moore P. Medication and substance abuse. In: Kryger M, Roth T, Dement W, eds. *Principles and Practices of Sleep Medicine.* 4th ed. Philadelphia: Saunders; 2005:1345–1358.

2. Patten CA, Choi WS, Gillin JC, Pierce JP. Depressive symptoms and cigarette smoking predict development and persistence of sleep problems in US adolescents. *Pediatrics.* 2000;106:E23.

3. Wong MM, Brower KJ, Zucker RA. Childhood sleep problems, early onset of substance use and behavioral problems in adolescence. *Sleep Med.* 2009;10:787–796.

4. Wong MM, Brower KJ, Fitzgerald HE, Zucker RA. Sleep problems in early childhood and early onset of alcohol and other drug use in adolescence. *Alcohol Clin Exp Res.* 2004;28:578–587.

5. Gregory AM, Caspi A, Eley TC, Moffitt TE, Oconnor TG, Poulton R. Prospective longitudinal associations between persistent sleep problems in childhood and anxiety and depression disorders in adulthood. *J Abnorm Child Psychol.* 2005;33:157–163.

6. Roberts RE, Roberts CR, Duong HT. Chronic insomnia and its negative consequences for health and functioning of adolescents: a 12-month prospective study. *J Adolesc Health.* 2008;42:294–302.

7. Roberts RE, Roberts CR, Chen IG. Impact of insomnia on future functioning of adolescents. *J Psychosom Res.* 2002;53:561–569.

8. Smith MT, Huang MI, Manber R. Cognitive behavior therapy for chronic insomnia occurring within the context of medical and psychiatric disorders. *Clin Psychol Rev.* 2005;25:559–592.

9. Jindal RD, Thase ME. Treatment of insomnia associated with clinical depression. *Sleep Med Rev.* 2004;8:19–30.

10. Deas D, Brown ES. Adolescent substance abuse and psychiatric comorbidities. J Clin Psychiatry. 2006;67:e02.

11. Sudsuang R, Chentanez V, Veluvan K. The effect of buddhist meditation on serum cortisol and total protein levels, blood pressure, pulse rate, lung volume and reaction time. *Physiol Behav.* 1991;50:543–548.

12. Carlson LE, Speca M, Faris P, Patel KD. One year pre-post intervention follow-up of psychological, immune, endocrine and blood pressure outcomes of mindfulness-based stress reduction (MBSR) in breast and prostate cancer outpatients. *Brain Behav Immun.* 2007;21:1038–1049.

13. Marcus M, Fine M, Moeller F, et al. Change in stress levels following mindfulness-based stress reduction in a therapeutic community. *Addict Dis Treat.* 2003;2:63–68.

14. Grossman P, Niemann L, Schmidt S, Walach H. Mindfulness-based stress reduction and health benefits. A meta-analysis. *J Psychosom Res.* 2004;57:35–43.

15. Jain S, Shapiro SL, Swanick S, et al. A randomized controlled trial of mindfulness meditation versus relaxation training: effects on distress, positive states of mind, rumination, and distraction. *Ann Behav Med.* 2007;33:11–21.

16. Witek-Janusek L, Albuquerque K, Chroniak KR, Chroniak C, Durazo-Arvizu R, Mathews HL. Effect of mindfulness based stress reduction on immune function, quality of life and coping in women newly diagnosed

with early stage breast cancer. *Brain Behav Immun.* 2008;22:969–981.

17. Teasdale JD, Segal ZV, Williams JM, Ridgeway V, Soulsby J, Lau M. Prevention of relapse/recurrence in major depression by mindfulness-based cognitive therapy. *J Consult Clin Psychol.* 2000;68:615–623.

18. Baer RA. Mindfulness training as a clinical intervention: a conceptual and empirical review. *Clin Psychol Sci Pract.* 2003;10:125–143.

19. Bootzin RR, Stevens SJ. Adolescents, substance abuse, and the treatment of insomnia and daytime sleepiness. *Clin Psychol Rev.* 2005;25:629–644.

20. Kaplan H, Goldenberg D, Galvin-Nadeau M. The impact of a meditation-based stress reduction program on fibromyalgia. Gen Hos Psychiatry. 1993;15:284–289.

21. Roth B, Robbins D. Mindfulness-based stress reduction and health-related quality of life: findings from a bilingual inner-city patient population. *Psychosom Med.* 2004;66:113–123.

22. Heidenreich T, Tuin I, Pflug B, Michal M, Michalak J. Mindfulness-based cognitive therapy for persistent insomnia: a pilot study. *Psychother Psychosom.* 2006;75:188–189.

23. Shapiro SL, Bootzin RR, Figueredo AJ, Lopez AM, Schwartz GE. The efficacy of mindfulness-based stress reduction in the treatment of sleep disturbance in women with breast cancer: an exploratory study. *J Psychosom Res.* 2003;54:85–91.

24. Carlson LE, Speca M, Patel KD, Goodey E. Mindfulness-based stress reduction in relation to quality of life, mood, symptoms of stress and levels of cortisol, dehydroepiandrosterone sulfate (DHEAS) and melatonin in breast and prostate cancer outpatients. *Psychoneuroendocrinology.* 2004;29:448–474.

25. Carlson LE, Garland SN. Impact of mindfulness-based stress reduction (MBSR) on sleep, mood, stress and fatigue symptoms in cancer outpatients. Int *J Behav Med.* 2005;12:278–285.

26. Goldenberg D, Kaplan K, Nadeau M, Brodeur C, Smith S, Schmid C. A controlled trial of a stress-reduction, cognitive behavioral treatment program in fibromyalgia. *J Muskuloskel Pain.* 1994;2:53–56.

27. Kreitzer MJ, Gross CR, Ye X, Russas V, Treesak C. Longitudinal impact of mindfulness meditation on illness burden in solid-organ transplant recipients. *Prog Transplant.* 2005;15:166–172.

28. Yook K, Lee SH, Ryu M, et al. Usefulness of mindfulness-based cognitive therapy for treating insomnia in patients with anxiety disorders: a pilot study. *J Nerv Ment Dis.* 2008;196:501–503.

29. Singh BB, Berman BM, Hadhazy VA, Creamer P. A pilot study of cognitive behavioral therapy in fibromyalgia. *Altern Ther Health Med.* 1998;4:67–70.

30. Bowen S, Witkiewitz K, Dillworth TM, et al. Mindfulness meditation and substance use in an incarcerated population. *Psychol of Addict Behav.* 2006;20:343–347.

31. Hoppes K. The application of mindfulness-based cognitive interventions in the treatment of co-occurring addictive and mood disorders. CNS Spectrum. 2006;11:829–851.

32. Marcus M, Fine M, Kouzekanani. Mindfulness-based meditation in a therapeutic community. *J Subst Abuse.* 2001;5:305–311.

33. Marcus MT, Schmitz J, Moeller G, et al. Mindfulness-based stress reduction in therapeutic community treatment: a stage 1 trial. Am *J Drug Alcohol Abuse.* 2009;35:103–108.

34. Zgierska A, Rabago D, Zuelsdorff M, Coe C, Miller M, Fleming M. Mindfulness meditation for alcohol relapse prevention: a feasibility pilot study. *J Addict Med.* 2008;2:165–173.

35. Breslin F, Zack M, McMain S. An information-processing analysis of mindfulness: implications for relapse prevention in the treatment of substance abuse. *Clin Psychol Sci Pract.* 2002;9:275–299.

36. Perlis ML, Jungquist C, Smith MT, et al. *Cognitive Behavior Therapy of Insomnia: A Session-By-Session Guide.* New York: Springer; 2005.

37. Kabat-Zinn J. *Full Catastophe Living: Using the Wisdom of Your Body and Mind to Face Stress, Pain and Illness.* New York: Delacorte Press; 1990.

38. Bootzin R, Shapiro S, Bailey E, Britton W. *Sleep Treatment Manual for Adolescents.* Tucson, AZ: University of Arizona; 2005.

39. Marlatt A. Addiction, mindfulness and acceptance. In: Hayes S, Jacobson N, Folette V, Dougher M, eds. *Acceptance and Change: Content and Context in Psychotherapy.* Reno, NV: Context Press; 1994:175–197.

40. Dennis M. *Global Appraisal of Individual Needs.* Version 1299. Bloomington, IN: Chestnut Health Systems; 1999.

41. Dennis ML, Dawud-Noursi S, Muck R, McDermeit MT. The need for developing and evaluating adolescent treatment models. In: Stevens SJ, Morral AR, eds. *Adolescent Drug Treatment in the United States: Exemplary Models from a National Evaluation Study.* Binghamton, NY: Haworth Press; 2003:3–34.

42. Dennis ML, Rourke KM, Lennox R, Campbell RS, Caddell JM. *Global Appraisal of Individual Needs: Background and Psychometric Properties Manual.* Research Triangle Park, NC: Research Triangle Institute; 1995.

43. Marlatt A, Gordon J. *Relapse Prevention.* New York: Guilford Press; 1985.

44. Needle R, Fisher D, Weatherby N. The reliability of self-reported HIV risk behaviors of drug users. Psychol Addict Behav. 1995;9:242–250.

45. NIDA. *Training Manual for Administering and Coding the Risk Behavior Assessment (RBA) Questionnaire.* Rockville, MD: Community Research Branch, National Institute on Drug Abuse, Alcohol, Drug Abuse, and Mental Health Administration; 1991.

46. Meyer TJ, Miller ML, Metzger RL, Borkovec TD. Development and validation of the Penn State Worry Questionnaire. *Behav Res Ther*. 1990;28:487–495.

47. Davey GC. A comparison of three worry questionnaires. *Behav Res Ther*. 1993;31:51–56.

48. Chorpita BF, Tracey SA, Brown TA, Collica TJ, Barlow DH. Assessment of worry in children and adolescents: an adaptation of the Penn State Worry Questionnaire. *Behav Res Ther*. 1997;35:569–581.

49. Behar E, Alcaine O, Zuellig AR, Barkovec TD. Screening for generalized anxiety disorder using the Penn State Worry Questionnaire: a receiver operating characteristic analysis. *J Behav Ther Exp Psychiatry*. 2003;34:25–43.

50. Bootzin RR, Engle-Friedman M. The assessment of insomnia. Behav Assess. 1981;3:107–126.

51. Haynes PL, Bootzin RR, Smith L, Cousins J, Cameron M, Stevens S. Sleep and aggression in substance-abusing adolescents: results from an integrative behavioral sleep-treatment pilot program. *Sleep*. 2006;29:512–520.

52. Johns MW. A new method for measuring daytime sleepiness: the Epworth sleepiness scale. *Sleep*. 1991;14:540–545.

53. Gibson ES, Powles AC, Thabane L, et al. "Sleepiness" is serious in adolescence: two surveys of 3235 Canadian students. BMC Public Health. 2006;6:116.

54. Stevens S, Haynes PL, Ruiz B, Bootzin RR. Effects of a behavioral sleep medicine intervention on trauma symptoms in adolescents recently treated for substance abuse. *Subst Abus*. 2007;28:21–31.

55. Harrison Y, Horne JA. The impact of sleep deprivation on decision making: a review. *J Exper Psychol Appl*. 2000;6:236–249.

56. Durmer JS, Dinges DF. Neurocognitive consequences of sleep deprivation. *Sem Neurol*. 2005;25:117–129.

57. Banks S, Dinges DF. Behavioral and physiological consequences of sleep restriction. *J Clin Sleep Med*. 2007;3:519–528.

58. Anderson C, Horne JA. Sleepiness enhances distraction during a monotonous task. *Sleep*. 2006;29:573–576.

59. Carmody J, Baer RA. Relationships between mindfulness practice and levels of mindfulness, medical and psychological symptoms and well-being in a mindfulness-based stress reduction program. *J Behav Med*. 2008;31:23–33.

60. Luders E, Toga A, Lepore N, Gaser C. The underlying anatomical correlates of long-term meditation: larger frontal and hippocampal volumes of gray matter. *Neuroimage*. 2009;45:672–678.

61. Lazar SW, Kerr CE, Wasserman RH, et al. Meditation experience is associated with increased cortical thickness. *Neuroreport*. 2005;16:1893–1897.

62. Lutz A, Greischar LL, Rawlings NB, Ricard M, Davidson RJ. Long-term meditators self-induce high-amplitude gamma synchrony during mental practice. *Proc Natl Acad Sci U S A*. 2004;101:16369–16373.

63. Brefczynski-Lewis JA, Lutz A, Schaefer HS, Levinson DB, Davidson RJ. Neural correlates of attentional expertise in long-term meditation practitioners. *Proc Natl Acad Sci U S A*. 2007;104:11483–11488.

64. Shapiro SL, Brown K, Biegel G. Teaching self-care to care-givers: effects of mindfulness-based stress reduction on mental health of therapists in training. *Training Educ Professional Psychol*. 2007;1:105–115.

65. Cahn BR, Polich J. Meditation (Vipassana) and the P3a event-related brain potential. Int *J Psychophysiol*. 2009;72:51–60.

66. Ong JC, Shapiro SL, Manber R. Mindfulness meditation and cognitive behavioral therapy for insomnia: a naturalistic 12-month follow-up. *Explore* (NY). 2009;5:30–36.

67. Ong JC, Shapiro SL, Manber R. Combining mindfulness meditation with cognitive-behavior therapy for insomnia: a treatment-development study. *Behav Ther*. 2008;39:171–182.

Psychosocial Treatment for Methamphetamine Use Disorders: A Preliminary Randomized Controlled Trial of Cognitive Behavior Therapy and Acceptance and Commitment Therapy

Matthew F. Smout, MPsych(Clin), PhD
Marie Longo, PhD
Sonia Harrison, MPsych(Clin)
Rinaldo Minniti, MPsych(Clin)
Wendy Wickes, MBBS
Jason M. White, PhD

ABSTRACT. Acceptance and Commitment Therapy (ACT) incorporates developments in behavior therapy, holds promise but has not been evaluated for methamphetamine use disorders. The objective of this study was to test whether ACT would increase treatment attendance and reduce methamphetamine use and related harms compared to cognitive behavior therapy (CBT). One hundred and four treatment-seeking adults with methamphetamine abuse or dependence were randomly assigned to receive 12 weekly 60-minute individual sessions of ACT or CBT. Attrition was 70% at 12 weeks and 86% at 24 weeks postentry. Per intention-to-treat analysis, there were no significant differences between the treatment groups in treatment attendance (median 3 sessions), and methamphetamine-related outcomes; however, methamphetamine use (toxicology-assessed and self-reported), negative consequences, and dependence severity significantly improved over time in both groups. Although ACT did not improve treatment outcomes or attendance compared to CBT, it may be a viable alternative to CBT for methamphetamine use disorders. Future rigorous research in this area seems warranted.

Matthew F. Smout is affiliated with the Centre for Treatment of Anxiety Disorders, Thebarton, South Australia, Australia.

Marie Longo is affiliated with School of Population Health, University of Queensland, Herston, Queensland.

Sonia Harrison, Rinaldo Minniti, and Wendy Wickes are affiliated with Drug and Alcohol Services South Australia, Warinilla Clinic, Norwood, South Australia, Australia.

Jason M. White is affiliated with the Discipline of Pharmacology, University of Adelaide, Adelaide, Australia.

The authors would like to thank Thomas Sullivan from DMAC, University of Adelaide, for his assistance with mixed models analyses.

This study was supported by the 2002 South Australian Premier's Drug Summit (Initiative R1.4 Young People and Amphetamines—Treatment).

INTRODUCTION

Methamphetamine use is associated with dependence (1), psychotic symptoms (2), depression (3), cognitive problems (4), unsafe sexual practices (5), and increased violence (6). All but one of the evaluations of psychotherapy for methamphetamine use disorders have been published in the last 5 years (7). Eight of the 12 studies have evaluated cognitive behavior therapy (CBT). The intensity of CBT protocols has ranged from 2 individual sessions (8, 9) to the Matrix program comprising 36 group CBT sessions plus adjunctive services (10). All interventions investigated led to reductions in methamphetamine use, including the comparison conditions, with brief CBT producing higher abstinence rates at 6-month follow-up than self-help (9), and the intensive Matrix program (11) producing higher abstinence rates than brief CBT. Attendance varied from an average of 26 from a possible 36 sessions attended in the Matrix program to 24% not attended in a 2-session CBT intervention, which may be attributable to sample characteristics (9, 11).

There have been a number of developments in CBT over the past 2 decades that have been largely untested in the treatment of substance use disorders. These include emphasizing observation of the thinking process rather than disputation and modification of thought content, reducing experiential avoidance through increasing distress tolerance (12) and acceptance skills (13), and values clarification to direct alternative activities to drug use (14, 15). Acceptance and Commitment Therapy (ACT) (13) incorporates all of the above developments.

To date only 2 published studies have investigated ACT as a treatment for substance use disorders. In a 3-arm randomized controlled trial, a comparison with Twelve Step Facilitation (TSF) therapy and methadone maintenance program alone for the treatment of methadone-maintained polysubstance-abusing clients, both ACT and TSF participants made comparable reductions in opiate and total drug use at the end of treatment. However, by 6-month follow-up, participants who received ACT, but not those who received TSF, achieved significantly lower opiate use than those treated with methadone

maintenance alone (16). Gifford and colleagues (17) randomly assigned cigarette smokers to receive nicotine-replacement therapy (NRT) plus medical management or ACT. Although quit rates were not different posttreatment, at 1-year follow-up those receiving ACT maintained their gains whereas a significantly higher proportion treated with NRT relapsed. Regarding ACT efficacy, comparisons between these 2 studies are limited because each study included a different sample and employed a different therapy format, with 32 1-hour individual sessions and 16 90-minute group sessions over 16 weeks in the former (16), and 7 50-minute individual sessions and 7 90-minute group sessions over 7 weeks in the latter (17).

The purpose of the present study was to test whether ACT might improve treatment outcomes or attendance in treatment-seeking adults with methamphetamine use disorders. To our knowledge, no clinical trial to date has assessed it in spite of anecdotal clinical success. Our primary hypotheses were that ACT would (1) reduce the amount of self-reported and objective (hair sample) methamphetamine use; (2) reduce self-reported severity of methamphetamine dependence and related negative consequences; and (3) increase treatment attendance compared to CBT. Our secondary hypotheses were that ACT would (1) improve self-reported symptom severity of depression, and physical and mental well-being; and (2) reduce self-reported and objective (hair sample) use of other drugs compared to CBT.

METHODS

Participants

Participants were primarily recruited from metropolitan outpatient (51% of total sample), inpatient (9%), and phone services (17%) of Drug and Alcohol Services South Australia between March 2004 and May 2006. Others were recruited through staff of and advertisements in health, community, and education services (e.g., vocational college and university campuses), independent magazines, newspapers, and radio

(16%) and referrals from clean needle programs (7%).

Eligible participants were between 16 and 65 years of age; met DSM-IV criteria for methamphetamine abuse or dependence according to the Mini-International Psychiatric Interview (MINI) substance use module (18), and methamphetamine was their drug of choice; reported average methamphetamine use of at least 2 days per week in the past 3 months; were willing to provide hair samples and maintain hair length at least 2 cm; and were available to attend appointments throughout the trial. Participants were *excluded* if in the past 8 weeks they reported having commenced or not maintained a stable dose of an antidepressant, antipsychotic or mood stabilizer medication; had a concurrent acute medical or psychiatric condition requiring hospitalization; or had a current medical or psychiatric condition that would prevent a clinical focus on psychotherapy for methamphetamine abuse (e.g., present suicidal intent) according to on-site medical officer assessment.

Of those screened, 12 were ineligible due to difficulties attending, insufficient amphetamine use or hair length, or unstable psychotropic medication regimens. One hundred and four people gave informed consent and were enrolled, underwent baseline assessment and subsequent randomization (see Figure 1). Ethics approval was obtained from the Human Research Ethics Committee of the University of Adelaide.

FIGURE 1. Participant flowchart.

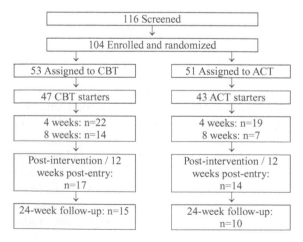

Interventions

Participants were randomly assigned to 12 weekly 60-minute individual sessions of CBT or ACT. This intensity of treatment was intended to provide greater therapeutic exposure than Baker et al.'s (19) 4-session protocol and achieve better adherence than the Matrix 36-session group protocol (20). Low attendances at past group treatments at our clinic dissuaded us from delivering interventions in groups.

Cognitive Behavior Therapy

The manual for this study encompassed Baker et al.'s (19) protocol supplemented with theoretical and procedural guidelines from Carroll (21). The most significant adaptation was that therapists individually tailored the timing and duration of CBT components following a treatment target hierarchy rather than session-specific outlines, as the fourth author's clinical experience suggested this could improve treatment attendance. The hierarchy consisted of maintaining rapport; enhancing motivation to minimize use; developing coping skills for *current* and a coping plan for *future* high-risk situations; education about apparently irrelevant decisions; long-term relapse prevention skills training; and CBT for other psychosocial problems that impact drug use. Whenever a higher target in the hierarchy was threatened, the therapists would redirect their attention from what they were covering to the higher treatment priority. Each session was structured in thirds: (1) review of drug use, cravings, and high-risk situations and homework exercises; (2) skill instruction and/or motivational interviewing (depending on progress); and (3) homework assignment and anticipation and development of a coping plan for high-risk situations.

Acceptance and Commitment Therapy

Hayes et al.'s (16) protocol was shortened from 32 to 12 sessions, and the manual provided additional guidance to therapists new to ACT. Session sequence was rearranged to begin with values clarification and valued activity scheduling, as this was considered a key mechanism by which ACT might impact methamphetamine abuse more powerfully than traditional CBT (22). Acceptance and defusion exercises were introduced to combat psychological barriers to enacting valued activities as they arose. Methamphetamine use was discussed primarily with a focus on how it interfered with performance of valued activities. Each session was structured in the following way: (1) mindfulness/acceptance exercise; (2) review of drug use and any significant events from the past week; (3) review of valued activity scheduling task; (4) introduction of a new core ACT skill; and (5) homework assignment (e.g., planning an action in service of value, mindfulness exercises).

The adapted CBT and ACT manuals are available from the authors upon request.

Therapists

Two therapists, a doctoral-level psychologist with 4 years' experience and a Masters-level psychologist with 1.5 years' experience, provided both ACT and CBT. They received 2 3-hour didactic training workshops in CBT from the fourth author (Masters-level psychologist with 20 years' experience), and a 4-day experiential and clinical skills workshop in ACT from an experienced ACT trainer. Eighty percent of participants gave written consent to having their sessions audio-recorded. Budgetary constraints precluded having audiotapes independently rated for adherence, but the tapes were reviewed during weekly supervision sessions for consistency with the manuals and enhancing treatment delivery (CBT sessions reviewed by fourth author; first and third authors reviewed each other's ACT sessions).

Outcome Measures

Self-reported methamphetamine use, negative consequences, and other drug use were assessed through a semistructured interview, conducted by the second author. This interview was developed for this study to allow descriptive information to be collected quickly (approximately 20 minutes) and in a format that could be interpreted straightforwardly (a copy of this instrument is available upon request). It had not been previously validated or pilot-tested.

The interview consisted of 6 sections: (1) time and amount of last methamphetamine use prior to interview; (2) demographic information; (3) medical, psychiatric, and drug use treatment history; (4) methamphetamine use history (mainly recent but including age at which at least monthly use started, and at which current route of administration started); (5) other drug use in past month; and (6) consequences of methamphetamine use.

Based on this interview, the primary outcome was the reported average amount of methamphetamine used in the past month; it was calculated by multiplying days used in previous month by the usual amount used per day, and reported in "points" ($\simeq 0.1$ g per "point"). Consequences of methamphetamine use included 17 items of this interview (e.g., slept too little, had an argument with someone) where clients reported the number of times each had occurred in previous month and 5 items (e.g., abscesses, infections, lost a friendship) rated dichotomously (yes $= 1$, no $= 0$). Responses were summed to form a negative consequences scale. In our study, this scale showed acceptable internal consistency (Cronbach $\alpha = .8$ at baseline) and criterion validity, demonstrated through moderate correlations with self-reported use (Pearson $r =$ .37, $P < .001$) and Leeds Dependence Questionnaire (see below) ($r = .44$, $P < .001$).

Objective methamphetamine and other drug use were determined by hair analysis. A 1 cm long segment of hair (50 to 100 hairs) was clipped from the scalp, representing approximately 1 month of growth. Hair samples were analyzed by Forensic Science SA. Amphetamine, methamphetamine, methylenedioxymethamphetamine (MDMA), diazepam, morphine, codeine, monoacetylmorphine, and diacetylmorphine concentrations were measured by high-performance liquid chromatography coupled with tandem mass spectrometry (LC/MS/MS) and provided quantitative information on substance use over the past month.

Severity of methamphetamine dependence was assessed using the Leeds Dependence Questionnaire (LDQ) (23). The LDQ consists of 10 psychological dependence symptoms (e.g., preoccupation, narrowed behavioral repertoire) rated for frequency on a 4-point scale (0 = never to 3 = nearly always). It has sound psychometric properties in outpatient populations including stimulant users (24).

Depression symptom severity was assessed using the Beck Depression Inventory (BDI-II) (25), the most widely used self-reported measure of depression and previously used in methamphetamine treatment outcome studies (9, 26). General mental health and physical health and well-being were assessed using the Short Form 12 (SF-12). Used in previous substance use research (27), it is a 12-item version of the extensively validated SF-36 questionnaire. SF-12 produces standard t-scores as a measure of these above-mentioned outcomes (28).

General motivational measures (Readiness to Change Questionnaire (29), Commitment to Abstinence Scale (30), and Worker Alliance Inventory short form (31)), therapy-specific measures (such as Acceptance and Action Questionnaire (32)), and unvalidated measures devised specifically for this study were also collected but there were too few data, due to study attrition, to conduct meaningful analyses, and so they are not reported here (see (33) for details).

The interview measuring self-reported methamphetamine use, related negative consequences, and other drug use was administered at baseline, after 4 and 8 therapy sessions, and 3 months posttreatment (4, 8, and 24 weeks postentry, respectively). Hair samples and the LDQ, BDI-II, and SF-12 data were collected at baseline and 12 and 24 weeks postentry. All measures were collected by 1 of 2 research assistants who were not blind to therapy assignment but did not provide treatment. Participants were reimbursed AUS$20 per assessment session completed.

Sample Size

Allowing for 40% attrition, and to have 80% power to detect a between-group difference effect size of Cohen's $d = 0.58$ based on the between-group difference in Baker and colleagues' study of methamphetamine users (8), the a priori estimated sample size was 128. An interim analysis after 2 years indicated the effect size and rate of recruitment were insufficient to demonstrate a between-group difference within the timeframe of the project's funding. Recruitment was discontinued after 104 participants had been enrolled. Already-enrolled participants were offered complete study intervention and assessments.

Randomization

An allocation table was constructed by dividing the estimated sample size into an equal number of clinician-therapy combinations. These were allocated to client ID via a computer-generated random number sequence. The second author then used this table to allocate participants; although the table was not concealed from the person assigning, it was not consulted other than at the time of randomization.

Statistical Methods

Descriptive statistics were analyzed using SPSS for Windows (version 13.0). Tests of the effects of psychotherapy condition on self-reported methamphetamine use, related negative consequences, and dependence, depression symptoms, health and well-being scores were analyzed using mixed effect models with SAS version 9.1 (SAS Institute, Cary, NC, USA) to estimate the missing 58% of the longitudinal data. Intent-to-treat analyses using separate models for each self-report outcome variable were tested, with therapy, time, and the interaction between therapy and time fitted as main effects and a random effect to account for correlations due to repeated measurements (34). This methodology provides unbiased estimates of the effect of treatment, assuming the data are missing at random and does not explicitly involve the imputation of missing data.

To correct for positive skewness, self-reported methamphetamine use and methamphetamine-related negative consequences scores were log transformed (ln function) with achieved normality. All other self-report variables were normally distributed. Objective methamphetamine data contained a large number of "zero" values and was non-normally distributed; therefore, it was dichotomized as hair positive (1) or negative (0) for methamphetamine, and analyzed using a logistic generalized estimating equation (GEE) regression model. Too many participants had "zero" hair concentrations of other drugs to allow a mixed effect or logistic GEE model analysis to compare interventions.

Significance level was set at 2-tailed P value $< .05$. Results are reported as mean $\pm$ standard deviation (SD) for normally distributed data, median (mdn) $\pm$ interquartile range (IQR) for skewed data or percentage/number, unless specified otherwise.

RESULTS

Participant Characteristics

Table 1 displays baseline characteristics for all participants ($N = 104$) enrolled in the trial. The majority were male, not working, injection drug users. Randomization appeared to be successful with no significant differences between CBT- and ACT-assigned participants on baseline measures.

Study Attrition and Treatment Attendance

Only 29.8% of those enrolled provided postintervention data (Figure 1). There were no significant differences in baseline characteristics between those who provided postintervention data and those who did not. "Weeks in study" (time between enrollment and final assessment or date of refusal to participate or failure to contact) was not significantly different between ACT and CBT groups (sample median 2.0 ± 12.8). Fourteen participants did not attend any treatment sessions, leaving 90 "treatment starters." There was no difference between CBT and ACT in treatment attendance: 61.1% of treatment starters attended at least 4 sessions (median 3.0 ± 5.5). There were no significant baseline differences on any demographic or outcome

TABLE 1. Baseline Characteristics of Enrolled Participants ($N = 104$)

Age, mean (SD)	30.9 years (6.5)
Female, %	40%
Education, %	25% 7–10 years
	49% 11–13 years
	17% Vocational education
	9% University
Current employment status, %	39% Unemployed
	39% Employed
	12% Student
	10% Other
Methamphetamine	
Number of days used in previous month, mean (SD)	16.1 (6.9)
Usual amount used in a day during previous month, median (IQR)	0.4 g (0.5)
Binged in last month, %	80.8%
Usual route of administration, %	
Injected	78%
Swallowed	14%
Snorted/smoked	8%
Total self-reported methamphetamine use in last month, median (IQR)	6.0 g (9.0)
Hair concentration methamphetamine, median (IQR)	1.95 ng/mg (4.58)
Methamphetamine-related negative consequences, mean (SD)	177.7 (66.6)
Leeds Dependence Questionnaire (LDQ) score, mean (SD)	18.6 (5.2)
Self-reported number of other drugs used in last month, mean (SD)	4.0 drugs (1.6)
Hair-analysis positive for at least one other drug (MDMA, codeine, morphine, diazepam, MAM) in last month,* %	29.8% positive for other drugs
Short Form 12 (SF-12)	47.6 (10.5)
Physical Health Composite Scale (PCS-12) score, mean (SD)	30.4 (8.9)
Mental Health Composite (MCS-12) score, mean (SD)	
Beck Depression Inventory (BDI-II) score, mean (SD)	26.8 (10.8)

*MDMA = 3,4-methylenedioxymethamphetamine; MAM = monoacetylmorphine.

TABLE 2. Comparison of Baseline ($N = 104$), Posttreatment (12 Weeks Postentry, $N = 31$), and Follow-Up (24 Weeks Postentry, $N = 25$) Outcome Measures

Outcome	CBT Baseline 12 weeks 24 weeks	ACT Baseline 12 weeks 24 weeks	Group x time interaction test	Time main effect test
Self-reported monthly total methamphetamine use (grams), median (IQR)	5.7 (9.3)	6.0 (7.0)	$F(4, 109) =$	$F(4, 109) = 49.31,$
	0.3 (1.0)	0.2 (3.0)	0.24,	$P < .01$
	0.4 (2.9)	0.8 (1.8)	$P = .92$	
Hair positive for methamphetamine, N (%)	51/53 (96.2%)	44/51 (86.3%)	$\chi^2(2) = 2.59,$	$\chi^{X2}(2) = 10.22,$
	8/14 (57.1%)	8/12 (66.7%)	$P = .27$	$P < .01$
	7/11 (63.6%)	4/8 (50%)		
Leeds Dependence Questionnaire (LDQ) scores, mean (SD)	18.2 (5.5)	19.0 (4.9)	$F(2, 51) = 0.02,$	$F(2, 51) = 60.56,$
	9.1 (8.0)	9.1 (6.8)	$p = .98$	$P < .01$
	9.3 (7.3)	10.1 (7.5)		
Methamphetamine-related negative consequences median (IQR)	107.0 (117.0)	103.0 (99.0)	$F(4, 107) = 0.82,$	$F(4, 107) = 42.98,$ $P < .01$
	15.0 (30.0)	12.0 (29.0)		
	4.5 (15.0)	6.0 (39.0)	$p = .52$	
Beck Depression Inventory (BDI-II) scores, mean (SD)	25.7 (11.2)	27.8 (10.3)	$F(2, 51) = 0.79,$	$F(2, 51) = 32.16,$
	17.7 (12.2)	15.4 (13.6)	$P = .46$	$P < .01$
	14.1 (14.8)	16.9 (16.3)		
Short Form 12 (SF-12) Physical Health Composite Scale (PCS-12), mean (SD)	48.5 (9.7)	46.7 (11.3)	$F(2, 52) = 1.73,$	$F(2, 52) = 0.47,$
	49.0 (9.1)	47.3 (10.8)	$p = .19$	$P = .63$
	52.9 (7.2)	44.7 (9.5)		
Short Form 12 (SF-12) Mental Health Composite Scale (MCS-12), mean (SD)	30.5 (9.7)	30.3 (8.1)	$F(2, 51) = 0.73,$	$F(2, 52) = 28.59,$
	40.8 (11.6)	44.3 (10.4)	$p = .49$	$P < .01$
	40.9 (15.4)	44.2 (12.7)		
Self-reported number of otherdrugs used in last month, mean (SD)	4.0 (1.5)	4.1 (1.7)	$F(4, 109) = 1.77,$	$F(4, 109) = 4.48,$
	3.4 (1.4)	3.6 (0.9)		$P < .01$
	3.1 (1.3)	3.4 (1.3)	$p = .14$	
Hair positive for at least one other drug, N (%)	17/53 (32.1%)	14/51 (27.5%)	$\chi^2(2) = 3.53,$	$\chi^{X2}(2) = 1.44,$
	3/14 (21.4%)	6/12 (50.0%)	$P = .17$	$P = .49$
	4/11 (36.4%)	4/8 (50.0%)		

Note. Group × time interaction and time main effects tested using mixed effect models, except hair positive for methamphetamine and hair positive for at least one other drug tested by logistic generalized estimating equation (GEE) regression models.

variable between those retained and lost at 12 and 24 weeks, respectively. Among those retained at 12 and 24 weeks, there were no significant differences between ACT and CBT groups.

Primary Outcome Analyses

Table 2 reports unadjusted means, medians, or frequencies for all outcome variables and results of mixed effect models tests. None of the main effects of therapy or therapy × time interactions were significant for any measure, but the main effect of time was significant for each measure. Post hoc comparisons revealed statistically significant within-group reductions in self-reported methamphetamine use, methamphetamine dependence, and negative consequences scores in both groups from baseline to 12 weeks postentry, without significant differences between the groups. Both groups had increased proportions of methamphetamine-free hair samples, too, but post hoc comparisons revealed that this change reached statistical significance for the CBT group only. There were no significant within-group changes between 12 and 24 weeks except for negative consequences, which further reduced significantly for CBT ($t(107) = 2.2$, $P = .03$), and showed only a trend toward improvement for ACT ($t(107) = 1.8$, $P = .08$).

Secondary Analyses

No therapy × time interactions were statistically significant for any secondary outcomes. There was a pre-post significant therapy effect for SF-12 physical scale scores only ($F(1, 52) = 4.81$, $P = .03$), favoring the CBT group (but without reaching statistical significance) at all time points. There was a significant main effect of therapy on depression and SF-12 mental health scores, and self-reported number of other drugs used (see Table 2). Post hoc comparisons revealed significant within-group reductions in depression and SF-12 mental health scale scores from baseline to 12 weeks for both CBT and ACT (without significant in-between group differences) and for self-reported number of other drugs for CBT only. There were no significant changes in any secondary measure from 12 to 24 weeks. Although side effect or adverse event data were not formally collected, none of the subjects reported any negative events during the study.

DISCUSSION

This study aimed to test whether ACT would improve treatment outcomes and attendance over conventional CBT in methamphetamine use disorders. The present ACT protocol did not achieve this. Participants in both ACT and CBT conditions showed comparable treatment attendance and reductions in self-reported methamphetamine use, related negative consequences, and dependence symptoms. Only the CBT group showed a significant improvement in objectively assessed methamphetamine use.

CBT recipients in this study achieved similar results to those in Baker et al. (9) who reported significant reductions in methamphetamine use, with abstinence rates between 40% and 50%. Considering treatment starters only ($N = 90$), the present attendance rate is similar to the 62%

rate for the CBT arm in Baker et al. study (9) where CBT was delivered as 4 60-minute individual sessions. On the other hand, present treatment attendance and abstinence rates were well short of those achieved in Matrix program, with its 36 90-minute group CBT sessions, adjunctive to other services (11). Sample characteristics may account for some of the differences in attendance and retention. The present sample, like Baker et al.'s (9), was predominantly male, unemployed, and using intravenous drugs, factors known to reduce attendance (35). By contrast, the Matrix sample was 55% female, 69% employed, and only a quarter used intravenous drugs. Nevertheless, the stark contrast between attendance experiences of the Matrix program and the Australian studies warrants further investigation.

This was the first empirical evaluation of ACT with a methamphetamine-abusing population, the first randomized controlled trial (RCT) of ACT in Australia, and the first to contrast ACT with CBT for substance use disorders. Consistent with previous studies (16, 17), ACT produced similar results to the comparison condition at posttreatment. Unlike previous studies, however, ACT did not produce superior outcomes at follow-up, although study attrition precluded an accurate investigation of this effect. Further research is needed to clarify whether this was due to the study population or inadequacies in the protocol or its execution.

Limitations

The study attrition rate was very high, resulting in large amount of missing data and, possibly, in the study being underpowered. Due to high attrition, the "effective" sample size was too small to allow for detection of nuanced differences in outcomes and prevented drawing final conclusions regarding treatment efficacy. This high attrition likely reflects some level of dissatisfaction with the treatment and suggests the need for revision of study protocols.

Nevertheless, the present study remains one of few RCTs in this field and retained some methodological strengths, including a large a priori sample size, use of intent-to-treat analyses, and objective drug concentration assessments.

Implications for Future Research

To date, ACT protocols for substance use disorders have relied on theoretical assumptions about the optimal sequence and spacing of intervention delivery. Future research should systematically address these components to determine whether they influence attendance (e.g., comparing protocols that begin with values clarification versus creative hopelessness). At least 2 broad directions seem worth pursuing in developing ACT interventions with predominantly injection-methamphetamine users. Given low attendance, future comparisons of ACT with CBT could combine each psychotherapy with a component known to enhance attendance, such as contingency management (26). It is possible that injection-methamphetamine users are willing to commit to brief therapy (4 sessions or less) only; therefore, ACT protocols could be adjusted to address each of its targeted processes within a shorter time frame.

CONCLUSIONS

The ACT protocol used in this RCT did not achieve greater reductions in self-reported or objective methamphetamine use, negative consequence, or dependence severity, and did not improve attendance compared to CBT among treatment-seeking adults with methamphetamine use disorders. However, ACT produced comparable results to CBT; although, due to study limitations, it is premature to draw firm conclusions about ACT treatment efficacy compared to CBT, ACT holds a promise for a treatment alternative for those affected by methamphetamine use disorders. Further work focused on ACT protocol development, treatment delivery, and efficacy seems warranted based on this study and given that existing treatments for methamphetamine use disorders still leave much room for improvement.

REFERENCES

1. Substance Abuse and Mental Health Services Administration Office of Applied Studies. *The NDSUH Report: Methamphetamine Use, Abuse and Dependence: 2002, 2003, and 2004*. Rockville, MD: Substance Abuse and Mental Health Services Administration; 2005.

2. McKetin R, McLaren J, Lubman DI, Hides L. The prevalence of psychotic symptoms among amphetamine users. *Addiction*. 2006;101:1473–1478.

3. Semple S, Patterson T, Grant I. Methamphetamine use and depressive symptoms among heterosexual men and women. *J Subst Use*. 2005;10:31–47.

4. Nordahl TE, Salo R, Leamon M. Neuropsychological effects of chronic methamphetamine use on neurotransmitters and cognition: a review. *J Neuropsychiat Clin Neurosci*. 2003;15:317–325.

5. Molitor F, Truax SR, Ruiz JD, Sun RK. Association of methamphetamine use during sex with risky sexual behaviors, and HIV infection among non-injection drug users. *West J Med*. 1998;168:93–97.

6. Wright S, Klee H. Violent crime, aggression and amphetamine: what are the implications for drug treatment services? *Drugs Edu Prev Pol*. 2001;8:73–90.

7. Lee NK, Rawson RA. A systematic review of cognitive and behavioural therapies for methamphetamine dependence. *Drug Alcohol Rev*. 2008;27:309–317.

8. Baker A, Boggs TG, Lewin TJ. Randomized controlled trial of brief cognitive-behavioural interventions among regular users of amphetamines. *Addiction*. 2001;96:1279–1287.

9. Baker A, Lee NK, Claire M, Lewin TJ, Grant T, Pohlman S, Saunders JB, Kay-Lambkin F, Constable P, Jenner L, Carr VJ. Brief cognitive-behavioural interventions for regular amphetamine users: a step in the right direction. *Addiction*. 2005;100:367–378.

10. Rawson RA, Gonzales R, Brethren P. Treatment of methamphetamine use disorders: an update. *J Subst Abuse Treat*. 2002;23:145–150.

11. Rawson RA, Marinelli-Casey P, Anglin MD, Dickow A, Frazier Y, Gallagher C, Galloway GP, Herrell J, Huber A, McCann MJ, Obert J, Pennell S, Reiber C, Vandersloot D, Zweben J, Methamphetamine Treatment Project Corporate Authors. A multi-site comparison of psychosocial approaches for the treatment of methamphetamine dependence. *Addiction*. 2004;99:708–717.

12. Linehan MM. *Cognitive Behavioral Treatment of Borderline Personality Disorder*. New York: Guilford; 1993.

13. Hayes SC, Strosahl KD, Wilson KG. *Acceptance and Commitment Therapy: An Experiential Approach to Behavior Change*. New York: Guilford; 1999.

14. Wagner CC, Sanchez FP. The role of values in motivational interviewing. In: Miller WR, Rollnick S, eds. *Motivational Interviewing: Preparing People for Change*, 2nd ed (pp. 284–298). New York: Guilford; 2002.

15. Wilson KG, Murrell AR. Values work in acceptance and commitment therapy: setting a course for behavioral treatment. In: Hayes SC, Follette VM, Linehan MM, eds. *Mindfulness and Acceptance: Expanding*

the Cognitive-Behavioral Tradition. New York: Guildford Press; 2004:120–151.

16. Hayes SC, Wilson KG, Gifford EV, Bissett R, Piasecki M. A preliminary trial of twelve-step facilitation and acceptance and commitment therapy with polysubstance-abusing methadone-maintained opiate addicts. *Behav Ther*. 2004;35:667–688.

17. Gifford EV, Kohlenberg BS, Hayes SC, et al. Acceptance-based treatment for smoking cessation. *Behav Ther*. 2004;35:689–705.

18. Sheehan DV, Lecrubier Y, Sheehan KH, et al. The Mini-International Neuropsychiatric Interview (M.I.N.I.): the development and validation of a structured diagnostic psychiatric interview for DSM-IV and ICD-10. J Clin Psychiat. 1998;59(Suppl 20):22–33.

19. Baker A, Kay-Lambkin F, Lee NK, Claire M, Jenner L. *A Brief Cognitive Behavioural Intervention for Regular Amphetamine Users*. Australian Government Department of Health and Ageing; 2003.

20. Obert JL, McCann MJ, Marinelli-Casey P, et al. The Matrix Model of outpatient stimulant abuse treatment: history and description. *J Psychoactive Drugs*. 2000;32:157–164.

21. Carroll KM. *Therapy Manuals for Addiction: A Cognitive-Behavioral Approach: Treating Cocaine Addiction*. Bethesda, MD: National Institute on Drug Abuse; 1998.

22. Wilson KG, Byrd MR. ACT for substance use and dependence. In: Hayes SC, Strosahl KD, eds. *A Practical Guide to Acceptance and Commitment Therapy* (pp. 153–184). New York: Springer; 2004.

23. Raistrick D, Bradshaw J, Tober G, Weiner J, Allison J, Healey C. Development of the Leeds Dependence Questionnaire (LDQ): a questionnaire to measure alcohol and opiate dependence in the context of a treatment evaluation package. *Addiction*. 1994;89:563–572.

24. Heather N, Raistrick D, Tober G, Godfrey C, Parrott S. Leeds dependence questionnaire: new data from a large sample of clinic attenders. *Addict Res Theory*. 2001;9:253–269.

25. Beck AT, Steer RA, Brown GK. *Manual for the BDI-II*. San Antonio, TX: Psychological Corporation; 1996.

26. Rawson RA, McCann MJ, Flammino F, et al. A comparison of contingency management and cognitive-behavioral approaches for stimulant-dependent individuals. *Addiction*. 2006;101:267–274.

27. Smith KW, Larson MJ. Quality of life assessments by adult substance abusers receiving publicly funded treatment in Massachusetts. *Am J Drug Alcohol Abuse*. 2003;29:323–335.

28. Ware JE, Kosinski M, Keller SD. A 12-item short-form health survey. *Med Care*. 1996;34:220–233.

29. Rollnick S, Heather N, Gold R, Hall W. Development of a short 'readiness to change' questionnaire for use in brief, opportunistic interventions among excessive drinkers. *Br J Addiction*. 1992;87:743–754.

30. Hall SM, Havassy BE. Commitment to abstinence and relapse to tobacco, alcohol, and opiates. In: Tims FM, Leukefeld CG, eds. Relapse and Recovery in Drug Abuse. Bethesda, MD: National Institute on Drug Abuse; 1986. NIDA Research Monograph 72.

31. Tracey TJ, Kokotovic AM. factor structure of the working alliance inventory. *Psychol Assess*. 1989;1:207–210.

32. Hayes SC, Strosahl KD, Wilson KG, et al. Measuring experiential avoidance: a preliminary test of a working model. *Psychol Record*. 2004;54:553–578.

33. Smout MF, Krasnikow S, Longo M, White JM. Psychotherapy for methamphetamine abuse: an empirical comparison between relapse prevention skills training and acceptance and commitment therapy. In: *The Amphetamine Treatment Project 2003–2007 Final Report*. Adelaide: Drug and Alcohol Services South Australia; 2007.

34. Gibbons RD, Hedeker D, Elkin I, et al. Some conceptual and statistical issues in analysis of longitudinal psychiatric data: application to the NIMH treatment of depression collaborative research program dataset. *Arch Gen Psychiatry*. 1993;50:739–750.

35. Maglione M, Chao B, Anglin MD. Correlates of outpatient drug treatment drop-out among methamphetamine users. *J Psychoactive Drugs*. 2004;32:221–228.

Development of an Acceptance-Based Coping Intervention for Alcohol Dependence Relapse Prevention

Cassandra Vieten, PhD
John A. Astin, PhD
Raymond Buscemi, PsyD
Gantt P. Galloway, PhD

ABSTRACT. Both psychological and neurobiological findings lend support to the long-standing clinical observation that negative affect is involved in the development and maintenance of alcohol dependence, and difficulty coping with negative affect is a common precipitant of relapse after treatment. Although many current approaches to relapse prevention emphasize change-based strategies for managing negative cognitions and affect, acceptance-based strategies for preventing relapse to alcohol use are intended to provide methods for coping with distress that are fundamentally different from, though in theory complementary to, approaches that emphasize control and change. This paper describes the development of Acceptance-Based Coping for Relapse Prevention (ABCRP), a new intervention for alcohol-dependent individuals who are within 6 months of having quit drinking. Results of preliminary testing indicate that the intervention is feasible with this population; and a small uncontrolled pilot study ($N = 23$) showed significant ($P < .01$) improvements in self-reported negative affect, emotional reactivity, perceived stress, positive affect, psychological well-being, and mindfulness level, as well as a trend ($P = .06$) toward reduction in craving severity between pre- and postintervention assessments. The authors conclude that this acceptance-based intervention seems feasible and holds promise for improving affect and reducing relapse in alcohol-dependent individuals, warranting further research.

INTRODUCTION

Numerous studies indicate that psychosocial distress and negative affect are associated with the development and maintenance of substance dependence (1–6). Negative affect is one of the most commonly cited reasons for relapse following treatment for alcohol dependence in

Cassandra Vieten, John A. Astin, Raymond Buscemi, and Gantt P. Galloway are affiliated with the California Pacific Medical Center Research Institute, San Francisco, California, USA.

The authors thank G. Alan Marlatt for his assistance during the design of the intervention, Henry Ohlhoff Programs for assisting with recruitment of participants, Warren Browner and California Pacific Medical Center Research Institute for ongoing support of this work, and the subjects for generously providing their time.

This project was made possible by grant number 1R21AA015398 from the National Institute for Alcohol Abuse and Alcoholism at the National Institutes of Health. Its contents are solely the responsibility of the authors and do not necessarily represent the official views of the National Institute for Alcohol Abuse and Alcoholism.

both adolescents and adults (7–11). The relationship between negative affect, addiction, and relapse has received additional empirical support from preclinical studies (12–17). For example, chronic stress appears to sensitize the brain reward system, rendering one more vulnerable to addiction (18). Drug-seeking may in part be explained by an affective downward spiral supported by negative reinforcement (relief of discomfort when drugs are taken), and a lower "hedonic set point" that reduces the efficacy of reinforcers, requiring increased intensity of use to maintain normal affect (19). Taken together, both psychological and neurobiological findings lend support to the long-standing clinical observation that people abuse alcohol and other substances despite serious consequences in part in order to regulate negative affect and cope with distress (20).

Reviews of the relapse prevention literature (21–23) provide support for the effectiveness of cognitive-behavioral therapy (CBT) approaches for relapse prevention in substance use disorders. Central to the CBT model of relapse is the identification of alcohol-related cues, potentially high-risk situations and relapse triggers—circumstances (e.g., people, places, events) in which an individual's efforts to refrain from alcohol use are threatened (24). Once there has been an assessment of the potential risks or triggers, the central task of CBT-based relapse prevention is to strengthen clients' capacity to cope more effectively with such situations by changing their approach to or level of engagement with these situations, and thereby reducing the risk of drinking behavior. CBT approaches to regulating negative affective states emphasize identifying and altering faulty cognitions that may lead to such states. Though CBT treatment and coping skills training have demonstrated considerable success in terms of helping individuals reduce the use of drugs and alcohol, a substantial proportion of treated individuals relapse (25, 26).

Our premise is that relapse prevention therapies could be enhanced by the inclusion of intervention components emphasizing acceptance. Although learning to avoid relapse triggers and controlling reactions to them using approaches such as "thought stopping" or cognitive reappraisal may be useful, the reality is that level of engagement with environmental cues cannot always be altered (e.g., exposure to billboards with alcohol advertisements, or family members with whom one used to drink alcohol), and cognitions and affective states cannot always be changed or controlled (27–29). Acceptance-based therapies may be complementary to traditional change-based CBT methods insofar as providing a set of skills directed specifically toward increasing *tolerance* of physiological, cognitive, and emotional distress or craving. This may improve the ability to regulate behavior, especially in situations where avoiding or changing cognitive-affective content is not possible.

Acceptance-based modalities may also provide an alternative and potentially more effective approach to regulating negative affect and craving than methods emphasizing change and control of internal relapse triggers (such as CBT). We have witnessed over the course of the past decade the emergence of what some have termed a "third-wave" of behavioral therapies that emphasize acceptance rather than control/change as the central component in the treatment of mood dysregulation. Recent developments within the field of CBT have led to a questioning of the mastery and control model that has historically characterized most CBT approaches to dealing with mood disturbance and addictive behaviors. This is evidenced in part by the growing clinical interest in and study of therapeutic modalities such as Dialectical Behavior Therapy (30), Acceptance and Commitment Therapy (31), Mindfulness-Based Stress Reduction (32), and Mindfulness-Based Cognitive Therapy (33), all of which emphasize acceptance of unwanted internal experiences as a core therapeutic component.

In contrast to traditional CBT where the emphasis is on altering maladaptive cognitions, moods, or behaviors, the focus in mindfulness- and acceptance-based interventions is on altering one's *relationship* to cognitive-emotional processes through the strengthening of a nonevaluative, metacognitive awareness (34). As noted by Baer (35), unlike most CBT methods, mindfulness does not involve the evaluation of cognitions as either rational or distorted, and does not attempt to change or dispute thoughts deemed to be irrational or maladaptive. Baer notes that, through mindfulness practice, one is instead taught to "observe thoughts, to note their impermanence, and to refrain from evaluating them."

The emphasis in many CBT approaches on avoidance/inhibition or alteration of negative cognitions and affective states may serve paradoxically to increase negative affect and maintain the association of negative affect with its cues (36–40). There is a growing body of experimental evidence suggesting that acceptance-based skills for coping with certain aversive experiences may actually be more effective than those emphasized by CBT. In a study of an anxiogenic stimulus (inhaled carbon dioxide), subjects employing mindful acceptance, when compared with individuals who attempted to control their experiences through the use of standard CBT techniques, reported less fear, appeared less behaviorally avoidant, and had fewer catastrophic thoughts during the noxious experience (41). Studies also suggest that the use of acceptance, as opposed to control/change-based strategies, can be more effective in helping subjects cope with laboratory induced pain (e.g., cold pressor test) (42, 43) and chronic pain (44). In alcoholics, evidence suggests that use of avoidant coping strategies predicts worse abstinence outcomes, (45) and that decreased cognitive avoidance and increased approach behaviors predict improved treatment outcomes (46).

Recent theoretical and empirical work by Marlatt and colleagues (47–51) suggests that mindfulness-based approaches may be effective for drug and alcohol use disorders. Compared to treatment-as-usual nonrandomized controls, incarcerated subjects who completed mindfulness training showed improvements on scales of impulse control, drug abuse severity, average weekly drug use, and drinking-related locus of control at 3-month follow-up. Subjects who received the mindfulness intervention also reported significant decreases in avoidance of thoughts when compared to controls, and this decrease partially mediated intervention effects on posttreatment alcohol use (52). Promising results of mindfulness-based interventions for smoking (53, 54) and eating disorders have been observed as well (55).

Studies suggest that Acceptance and Commitment Therapy (ACT) (31) may be a potentially effective treatment for addictive disorders (56–58). ACT stresses the development of greater "acceptance," which is defined as being "experientially open" to the reality of the present moment, and incorporates mindfulness exercises as part of its therapeutic approach. In a randomized trial with polysubstance abusing opiate addicts enrolled in a methadone maintenance program, those who received the ACT intervention evidenced a greater decrease in opiate use than "standard of care" or 12-step groups (57). A trial by Gifford found that among smokers, those receiving ACT exhibited significantly better smoking outcomes at 1-year follow-up when compared to those receiving nicotine replacement therapy, and that those outcomes were mediated by acceptance-related skills (58).

In summary, although traditional approaches to relapse prevention emphasize change-based strategies for reducing and managing stress and negative affect, these approaches are only partially effective and relapse continues to be a challenge. Our hypothesis was that an acceptance-based approach, based upon training in mindfulness, would improve outcomes in treated alcoholics by providing new skills for affect regulation that are different from, though in theory complementary to, traditional CBT approaches.

The goal of the present study was to develop and pilot test an acceptance-based relapse prevention intervention directed toward reducing relapse and improving affect regulation and psychological well-being in alcohol-dependent individuals who have recently quit drinking.

METHODS

Intervention Development

The first 3 months of the project were devoted to the development of a provisional manual for the Acceptance-Based Coping for Relapse Prevention (ABCRP) intervention. This process started with a review of the literature on mindfulness- and acceptance-based interventions for behavioral, mood and anxiety disorders, negative affect, affect regulation, coping, and predictors of both relapse and successful treatment response. The intervention was developed using a "problem formulation" approach (59) that calls for tailoring interventions to match the targeted population and problems. We detailed the symptoms we hoped to alleviate, as well as the skills we hoped to enhance with the intervention, and then selected or developed intervention components that would address each of these problems. In addition, we consulted with other groups developing mindfulness interventions for substance abuse and behavioral disorders. This intervention drew upon several mindfulness- and acceptance-based interventions: Mindfulness-Based Stress Reduction (32), Mindfulness-Based Cognitive Therapy (33), Mindfulness-Based Relapse Prevention (50), and Acceptance and Commitment Therapy (60). Through an iterative process of revisions among investigators and consultants, we developed a provisional ABCRP treatment manual, which focused on mindfulness training and applications of acceptance-based coping for managing stress, craving, and negative affect.

Several elements distinguish our protocol from other, above-mentioned, mindfulness-based therapies. Whereas the development of more focused attention and the skills of observation and concentration are central to most mindfulness-based interventions, our protocol emphasized cultivation of nonresistance to, non-avoidance of, and capacity to tolerate and even explore one's internal states (e.g., thoughts, feelings, sensations), rather than the development of greater control over one's attentional faculties. In addition, rather than viewing acceptance strictly as a skill one must train and develop, the ABCRP intervention emphasized discovery of, and increasing familiarity with, one's natural capacity for experiential openness and nonresistance to challenging mental-emotional states as inherent qualities of awareness itself. Based on the theory that relapse is in part the result of an individual's efforts to manage or control unwanted internal experiences, we hypothesized that increasing one's willingness, capacity, and self-efficacy to experience (i.e., accept) stress, craving, and negative affect, rather than reflexively attempting to avoid, change, or control these states, would reduce the likelihood of relapse.

The intervention consisted of 8 weekly 2-hour group-based sessions and a follow-up "booster"

session 4 weeks later. Groups took place in an urban hospital and were facilitated by the first 2 authors—a licensed clinical psychologist with experience in addiction treatment and a health psychologist, both experienced in delivering mindfulness-based interventions. The following topics constituted the central focus of the 8-week intervention: (1) introduction to the concept of mindfulness and its potential to impact one's relationship to the experience of unwanted internal experiences (including stress and craving) that are frequent precipitants of alcohol relapse; (2) the attitudinal foundations of mindful awareness (i.e., learning to observe internal and external experiences with the qualities of acceptance/nonjudgment, curiosity, openness, and nonstriving; (3) cultivation of greater willingness to experience rather than avoid or attempt to alter distressing mental-emotional states, with the intention of making such states more manageable and less aversive; (4) gaining familiarity with the "observing self," or the capacity to be "metacognitively" and "nonreactively" aware of one's own internal affective states and mental perspectives, with the intention of having greater understanding, and, thus, freedom of behavioral choice in response to such states; and (5) gaining greater objectivity in relationship to one's own mental processes, i.e., being able to recognize that thoughts are not necessarily accurate representations of self or reality.

Feasibility

Following the 3-month intervention development phase, over the next 6 months, we tested the feasibility of the provisional ABCRP intervention in 2 consecutive cohorts of 22 individuals participating in a local substance abuse treatment program.

Based on participant feedback as well as weekly discussion among the research team, the intervention manual was refined. Changes included reducing the length of weekly sessions from 2 hours to 90 minutes; shortening the length of in-class meditation sessions; and incorporating more direct links between the taught mindfulness skills and relapse prevention, particularly in terms of applying the skills of mindful acceptance on a day-to-day basis to common relapse triggers of craving and negative affect. Another important change was the inclusion of additional, between-session contact with participants, in the form of weekly e-mails or letters. These communiqués served as a reinforcement of what was discussed in the prior-week class, and of the mindfulness and acceptance skills by bringing additional attention to them. Feedback from participants who underwent the revised study intervention indicated that these additional contacts were very helpful, and appeared anecdotally to enhance treatment retention and adherence.

Following this 6-month period of manual refinement, we pilot-tested, over the course of 1 year, the developed ABCRP intervention using 3 consecutive cohorts of individuals participating in a local substance abuse treatment program. Pilot-level findings on feasibility and efficacy of ABCRP intervention, based on these 3 cohorts ($N = 33$), are presented in this article.

Recruitment

Study participants were recruited from the general community as well as from local treatment centers, 12-step programs, and physicians' offices. Eligible participants were English-speaking adults over the age of 18, in their first 6 months of having quit drinking, and who meet the ICD-10 screening criteria for alcohol dependence. Exclusion criteria were a self-reported history of psychiatric disorders involving hallucinations or delusions. This study was approved by the Institutional Review Board of California Pacific Medical Center prior to any procedures.

Measures

Negative affect was assessed using the Positive and Negative Affect Scale (PANAS) (61), a 20-item questionnaire measuring the degree to which the respondent experienced positive affect (e.g., active, enthusiastic, inspired) or negative affect (e.g., afraid, irritable, distressed) over a specified time period on a scale from 1 (slightly or not at all) to 5 (extremely). Good reliability has been demonstrated in both subscales (Cronbach alpha = 0.85–0.89) (62). Subjects'

appraisals of their degree of life stress was assessed using the Perceived Stress Scale (PSS) (63), a 10-item measure that is the most widely used psychological instrument for measuring the perception of stress, with well-established internal consistency (alpha = .78) and reliability ($r = .85$). Craving or urge for an alcoholic drink was measured using the 8-item Alcohol Urge Questionnaire (AUQ) (64), which has demonstrated high internal consistency (0.91), retest reliability (1-day acute craving complete interval, 0.82), and good construct validity evidenced by strong correlations with measures of alcohol dependence severity (64). Overall psychological well-being was assessed using the Psychological General Well-Being Index (PGWBI), a 22-item measure of subjective well-being (65) that has demonstrated validity and reliability in numerous studies (66). Emotional reactivity was measured using a subscale of the investigator-developed Affect Regulation Measure (ARM), a 72-item scale measuring affect tolerance, cognitive regulation, discharge, preoccupation, somaticization, emotional reactivity, and lability. This measure demonstrates good internal consistency (alpha = .87), Rasch person separation reliabilities (Person $R = .89$), and test-retest reliabilities over 8 weeks of .84. Mindfulness was assessed using the brief Five-Factor Mindfulness Questionnaire (67), a 23-item measure that assesses 5 distinct but intercorrelated facets of mindfulness, including the capacity to observe and describe one's state, nonreactivity, nonjudgmentalness, and the capacity to act with greater awareness/attention, with strong concurrent validity and internal consistencies ranging from .72 to .92. At each time point, percent days abstinent served as our primary alcohol use outcome and was assessed using Timeline Follow Back Method (TLFB) (68) for the previous 3 months. The TLFB has been shown to be reliable ($r = .77–.90$) when administered by phone (69).

All measures were administered via Web-based survey software (questionnaires) or telephone (TLFB) prior to participation in the intervention, following the 8-week intervention (between 9 and 12 weeks postentry, prior the 4-week postintervention booster session), and 6 months postentry.

Statistical Analysis

SPSS for Windows version 13 statistical software was used for data analysis. An examination of histograms indicated that data were normally distributed. Subjects from the last three cohorts who completed the study intervention ($N = 23$) were included in the analysis. Using paired t tests, baseline and postintervention data were compared for psychological outcomes, and postintervention and 6 months postenrollment data for drinking outcomes (percent days abstinent) were compared. Significance level was set at .05, 2-tailed. Data are presented as mean (standard deviation, SD) unless otherwise specified.

RESULTS

Sample Characteristics

Women constituted 39% of the sample ($N = 33$), the mean age was 45 (SD = 7.2); 29% were 25 to 40 years old, 58% were 40 to 55, and 13% were over 55 years of age. Eighty percent were Caucasian, 10% Hispanic, 3% African American, 3% Asian, 3% other. Just over half of the sample (55%) was single, 39% were married or had a long-term partner, and 6% were divorced, separated, or widowed.

Attendance and Attrition

Ten out of 33 individuals failed to complete the intervention, defined as attendance at less than 50% of the 8 sessions, and were lost to follow-up. Among these 10 noncompleters, 3 attended no classes, 5 attended 1 class, and 2 attended 2 classes; 5 were in the first, 3 in the second, and 2 in the third cohort, suggesting an improved retention, possibly due to refinement of the intervention and study methods. At 6 months postenrollment, 18 of the 23 study completers provided data, the remaining 5 subjects were lost to follow-up.

Results

Paired-samples t tests of data of study completers ($N = 23$), collected pre- and postintervention, indicated positive changes in level of the following variables: craving (decrease of 32%;

$P = .06$); positive affect (increase of 20%; $P = .004$); negative affect (decrease of 32%; $P = .0001$); emotional reactivity (decrease of 17%; $P = .0001$); psychological well-being (increase of 15%; $P = .004$); perceived stress (decrease of 23%; $P = .002$); and mindfulness (increase of 21%; $P = .002$).

At postintervention, study completers ($N = 23$) reported mean percent days abstinent of 97.6 (10.1). At 6 months postenrollment ($N =18$), percent days abstinent decreased to 87.5 (21.5), but this change was not statistically significant. During the study, no side effects or adverse events were reported.

DISCUSSION

The goals of the project were to develop an acceptance-based intervention targeted toward preventing relapse in alcohol-dependent individuals attempting to quit drinking, and to pilot-test the feasibility and potential effectiveness of the intervention. Our preliminary findings suggest that Acceptance-Based Relapse Prevention holds promise for preventing alcohol relapse, and improving mood, emotional reactivity, and levels of craving, negative affect, positive affect, and mindfulness, and warrants further research. The promise of mindfulness-based interventions for relapse prevention is supported by similar research by Zgierska et al. (70) who conducted a small pilot study using a similar intervention in alcohol-dependent adults and found similar results.

Mindfulness- and acceptance-based treatments challenge traditional notions of affect regulation in that they focus on allowing distressing cognitions and affective states to remain as they are, rather than working to alter or change their content. A relatively recent addition to some CBT relapse prevention models, "urge surfing," has some similarity to a mindfulness/acceptance perspective, but is part of a comprehensive treatment approach, and its impact alone has not yet been studied. Twelve-step–based programs have long recommended "acceptance," embedded in a highly structured spiritual and social context, as the primary strategy for approaching negative affect and difficult life circumstances.

But most conceptualizations of emotion regulation rest upon the premise that negative affect needs to be controlled, managed, or regulated, and emotion regulation is often construed as the processes by which one decreases negative affect and increases positive affect.

However, as we have reviewed, exactly the same motivational process (e.g., the desire to reduce negative affect and increase positive affect) is involved in addiction. It may be that a more adaptive form of affect regulation would enhance the capacity to tolerate negative affect without necessarily decreasing it, and would allow to derive reward from positive affect without needing to enhance it, and would facilitate experience of mental-emotional states without reflexively feeling driven by conditioning to act upon them.

The extent to which acceptance- and mindfulness-based therapies are compatible and overlap with traditional CBT approaches remains to be seen. In treating addiction and preventing relapse, it may be equally useful to (1) acquire skills to identify and avoid relapse triggers and change thoughts that may lead to relapse, and (2) to increase tolerance for difficult cognitions, emotions, and craving states through acceptance. However, it may be difficult to discern which skill is needed at what times, and although the approaches may be complementary, they also differ from one another.

In this formative work, we developed and refined an acceptance-based intervention for relapse prevention (manual available from the authors upon request) that can be used in combination with or in addition to other treatment modalities. We have shown that teaching acceptance-based coping appears to be feasible in a mixed treatment for alcoholics who have quit drinking within the past 6 months.

Our findings should be interpreted as preliminary support for the potential clinical promise of this intervention because they are limited by several factors, including lack of a control group, small sample size, high attrition, and lack of an intent-to-treat analysis. Future studies should test acceptance-based interventions in adequately powered controlled trials, and explore further whether acceptance-based strategies are more effective than change-based strategies for relapse prevention in alcohol-dependent individuals in early recovery.

REFERENCES

1. Brewer DD, Catalano RF, Haggerty K, Gainey RR, Fleming CB. A meta-analysis of predictors of continued drug use during and after treatment for opiate addiction. *Addiction.* 1998;93:73–92.

2. Brady KT, Sonne SC. The role of stress in alcohol use, alcoholism treatment, and relapse. *Alcohol Res Health.* 1999;23:263–271.

3. Brown SA, Vik PW, Patterson TL, Grant I, Schuckit MA. Stress, vulnerability and adult alcohol relapse. *J Stud Alcohol.* 1995;56:538–545.

4. Carmody TP. Preventing relapse in the treatment of nicotine addiction: current issues and future directions. *J Psychoactive Drugs.* 1992;24:131–158.

5. Lowman C, Allen J, Stout RL. Replication and extension of Marlatt's taxonomy of relapse precipitants: overview of procedures and results. The Relapse Research Group. *Addiction.* 1996;91(Suppl):S51–S71.

6. Schmidt NB, Buckner JD, Keough ME. Anxiety sensitivity as a prospective predictor of alcohol use disorders. *Behav Modif.* 2007;31:202–219.

7. Brown SA. Recovery patterns in adolescent substance abuse. In: Baer JS, Marlatt GA, McMahon RJ, eds. *Addictive Behaviors Across the Life Span.* London: Sage; 1993:160–183.

8. Cornelius JR, Maisto SA, Pollock NK, et al. Rapid relapse generally follows treatment for substance use disorders among adolescents. *Addict Behav.* 2003;28:381–386.

9. Ciraulo DA, Piechniczek-Buczek J, Iscan EN. Outcome predictors in substance use disorders. *Psychiatr Clin North Am.* 2003;26:381–409.

10. Hodgins DC, el-Guebaly N, Armstrong S. Prospective and retrospective reports of mood states before relapse to substance use. *J Consult Clin Psychol.* 1995;63:400–407.

11. Zywiak WH, Westerberg VS, Connors GJ, Maisto SA. Exploratory findings from the Reasons for Drinking Questionnaire. *J Subst Abuse Treat.* 2003;25:287–292.

12. Goeders NE. Stress and cocaine addiction. *J Pharmacol Exp Ther.* 2002;301:785–789.

13. Koob GF, Le Moal M. Drug addiction, dysregulation of reward, and allostasis. *Neuropsychopharmacology.* 2001;24:97–129.

14. Abbot NC, Stead LF, White AR, Barnes J, Ernst E. Hypnotherapy for smoking cessation. *Cochrane Database Syst Rev.* 2000(2):CD001008.

15. Lyvers M. "Loss of control" in alcoholism and drug addiction: a neuroscientific interpretation. *Exp Clin Psychopharmacol.* 2000;8:225–249.

16. Sinha R. How does stress increase risk of drug abuse and relapse? *Psychopharmacology (Berl).* 2001;158:343–359.

17. Will MJ, Watkins LR, Maier SF. Uncontrollable stress potentiates morphine's rewarding properties. *Pharmacol Biochem Behav.* 1998;60:655–664.

18. Marinelli M, Piazza PV. Interaction between glucocorticoid hormones, stress and psychostimulant drugs. *Eur J Neurosci.* 2002;16:387–394.

19. Koob GF, Le Moal M. Drug abuse: hedonic homeostatic dysregulation. *Science.* 1997;278:52–58.

20. Carpenter KM, Hasin D. A prospective evaluation of the relationship between reasons for drinking and DSM-IV alcohol-use disorders. *Addict Behav.* 1998;23:41–46.

21. Caroll KM. Relapse prevention as a psychosocial treatment: a review of controlled clinical trials. *Exp Clin Psychopharmacol.* 1996;4:46–54.

22. Irvin JE, Bowers CA, Dunn ME, Wang MC. Efficacy of relapse prevention: a meta-analytic review. *J Consult Clin Psychol.* 1999;67:563–570.

23. Miller WR, Wilbourne PL. Mesa Grande: a methodological analysis of clinical trials of treatments for alcohol use disorders. *Addiction.* 2002;97:265–277.

24. Witkiewitz K, Marlatt GA. Relapse prevention for alcohol and drug problems: that was Zen, this is Tao. *Am Psychol.* 2004;59:224–235.

25. Project MATCH RG. Matching alcoholism treatments to client heterogeneity: project MATCH posttreatment drinking outcomes. *J Stud Alcohol.* 1997;58:7–29.

26. Rawson RA, Marinelli-Casey P, Anglin MD, et al. A multi-site comparison of psychosocial approaches for the treatment of methamphetamine dependence. *Addiction.* 2004;99:708–717.

27. Astin JA, Anton-Culver H, Schwartz CE, et al. Sense of control and adjustment to breast cancer: the importance of balancing control coping styles. *Behav Med.* 1999;25:101–109.

28. Astin JA, Shapiro SL, Schwartz CE, Shapiro DH. "The courage to change and the serenity to accept"— Further comments on fighting spirit and breast cancer. *Adv Mind Body Med.* 2001;17:142–144; discussion 145–146.

29. Carmody TP, Vieten C, Astin JA. Negative affect, emotional acceptance, and smoking cessation. *J Psychoactive Drugs.* 2007;39:499–508.

30. Linehan MM. Dialectical behavior therapy for treatment of borderline personality disorder: implications for the treatment of substance abuse. *NIDA Res Monogr.* 1993;137:201–216.

31. Hayes SC, Strosahl K, Wilson KG. *Acceptance and Commitment Therapy: An Experiential Approach to Behavior Change.* New York: Guilford; 1999.

32. Kabat-Zinn J. An outpatient program in behavioral medicine for chronic pain patients based on the practice of mindfulness meditation: theoretical considerations and preliminary results. *Gen Hosp Psychiatry.* 1982;4:33–47.

33. Segal Z, Williams M, Teasdale JD. *Mindfulness-Based Cognitive Therapy for Depression: A New Approach to Preventing Relapse.* New York: Guilford Press; 2002.

34. Teasdale JD, Moore RG, Hayhurst H, Pope M, Williams S, Segal ZV. Metacognitive awareness and prevention of relapse in depression: empirical evidence. *J Consult Clin Psychol.* 2002;70:275–287.

35. Baer RA. Mindfulness training as a clinical intervention: a conceptual and empirical review. *Clin Psychol Sci Pract.* 2003;10:125–143.

36. Blackledge JT, Hayes SC. Emotion regulation in acceptance and commitment therapy. *J Clin Psychol.* 2001;57:243–255.

37. Craske MG, Rowe M, Lewin M, Noriega-Dimitri R. Interoceptive exposure versus breathing retraining within cognitive-behavioural therapy for panic disorder with agoraphobia. *Br J Clin Psychol.* 1997;36:85–99.

38. Wegner DM. Ironic processes of mental control. *Psychol Rev.* 1994;101:34–52.

39. Wegner DM, Zanakos SI. Chronic thought suppression. *J Person.* 1994;62:615–640.

40. Forsyth JP, Barrios V, Acheson DT. Exposure therapy and cognitive interventions for the anxiety disorders: overview and newer third-generation perspectives. In: Richard DCS, Lauterbach D, eds. *Handbook of Exposure Therapies.* New York: Academic Press; 2006.

41. Eifert GH, Heffner M. The effects of acceptance versus control contexts on avoidance of panic-related symptoms. *J Behav Ther Exp Psychiatry.* 2003;34:293–312.

42. Keogh E, Bond FW, Hanmer R, Tilston J. Comparing acceptance- and control-based coping instructions on the cold-pressor pain experiences of healthy men and women. *Eur J Pain.* 2005;9:591–598.

43. Feldner MT, Hekmat H, Zvolensky MJ, Vowles KE, Secrist Z, Leen-Feldner EW. The role of experiential avoidance in acute pain tolerance: a laboratory test. *J Behav Ther Exp Psychiatry.* 2006;37:146–158.

44. McCracken LM, Eccleston C. Coping or acceptance: what to do about chronic pain? *Pain.* 2003;105:197–204.

45. Moser AE, Annis HM. The role of coping in relapse crisis outcome: a prospective study of treated alcoholics. *Addiction.* 1996;91:1101–1113.

46. Chung T, Langenbucher J, Labouvie E, Pandina RJ, Moos R. Changes in alcoholic patients' coping response predict 12-month treatment outcomes. *J Consult Clin Psychol.* 2001;69:92–100.

47. Marlatt GA. Buddhist philosophy and the treatment of addictive behavior. *Cogn Behav Pract.* 2002;9:44–49.

48. Marlatt GA. Mindfulness and metaphor in relapse prevention: an interview with G. Alan Marlatt. Interview by Deborah K. Shattuck. *J Am Diet Assoc.* 1994;94:846–848.

49. Marlatt GA, Kristeller JL. Mindfulness and meditation. In: Miller WR, ed. *Integrating Spirituality Into Treatment: Resources for Practitioners.* Washington, DC: American Psychological Association; 1999:67–84.

50. Witkiewitz K, Marlatt GA, Walker DE. Mindfulness-based relapse prevention for alcohol and substance use

disorders: the meditative tortoise wins the race. *J Cogn Psychother.* 2005;19:211–228.

51. Bowen S, Witkiewitz K, Dillworth TM, et al. Mindfulness meditation and substance use in an incarcerated population. *Psychol Addict Behav.* 2006;20:343–347.

52. Bowen S, Witkiewitz K, Dillworth TM, Marlatt GA. The role of thought suppression in the relationship between mindfulness meditation and alcohol use. *Addict Behav.* 2007;32:2324–2328.

53. Davis JM, Fleming MF, Bonus KA, Baker TB. A pilot study on mindfulness based stress reduction for smokers. *BMC Complement Altern Med.* 2007;7:2.

54. Michalsen A, Richarz B, Reichardt H, et al. [Smoking cessation for hospital staff. A controlled intervention study]. *Dtsch Med Wochenschr.* 2002;127:1742–1747.

55. Kristeller J, Hellet CB. An exploratory study of a mediation-based intervention for binge eating disorder. *J Health Psychol.* 1999;4:357–363.

56. Hayes SC, Wilson KG, Gifford E, et al. The use of Acceptance and Commitment Therapy and 12-step facilitation in the treatment of polysubstance abusing heroin addicts on methadone maintenance: a randomized controlled trial. Paper presented at Association of Behavior Analysis meeting; 2002; Toronto.

57. Bissett RT. *Processes of Change: Acceptance Versus 12-Step in Polysubstance Abusing Methadone Clients.* University of Nevada; 2001.

58. Gifford E. Acceptance-based treatment for smoking cessation. *Behav Ther.* 2004;35:689–705.

59. Teasdale JD, Segal Z, Williams M. Mindfulness training and problem formulation. *Clin Psychol Sci Pract.* 2003;10:157.

60. Hayes SC, Luoma JB, Bond FW, Masuda A, Lillis J. Acceptance and commitment therapy: model, processes and outcomes. *Behav Res Ther.* 2006;44:1–25.

61. Watson D, Clark LA, Tellegen A. Development and validation of brief measures of positive and negative affect: the PANAS scales. *J Person Soc Psychol.* 1988;54:1063–1070.

62. Crawford JR, Henry JD. The positive and negative affect schedule (PANAS): construct validity, measurement properties and normative data in a large non-clinical sample. *Br J Clin Psychol.* 2004;43(Pt 3):245–265.

63. Cohen S, Williamson G. Perceived stress in a probability sample of the United States. In: Spacapan S, Oskamp S, eds. *The Social Psychology of Health: Claremont Symposium on Applied Social Psychology.* Newbury Park, CA: Sage; 1988.

64. Bohn MJ, Krahn DD, Staehler BA. Development and initial validation of a measure of drinking urges in abstinent alcoholics. *Alcohol Clin Exp Res.* 1995;19:600–606.

65. Dupuy HJ. The Psychological General Well-Being (PGWB) Index. In: Wenger NK, Mattson ME, eds. *Assessment of Quality of Life in Clinical Trials of Cardiovascular Therapies.* Le Jacq Publishing; 1984:353–356.

66. Revicki DA, Leidy NK, Howland L. Evaluating the psychometric characteristics of the Psychological General Well-Being Index with a new response scale. *Qual Life Res.* 1996;5:419–425.

67. Baer RA, Smith GT, Hopkins J, Krietemeyer J, Toney L. Using self-report assessment methods to explore facets of mindfulness. *Assessment.* 2006;13:27–45.

68. Sobell LC, Sobell MB, Connors GJ, Agrawal S. Assessing drinking outcomes in alcohol treatment efficacy studies: selecting a yardstick of success. *Alcohol Clin Exp Res.* 2003;27:1661–1666.

69. Sobell LC, Brown J, Leo GI, Sobell MB. The reliability of the Alcohol Timeline Followback when administered by telephone and by computer. *Drug Alcohol Depend.* 1996;42:49–54.

70. Zgierska A, Rabago D, Zuelsdorff M, Coe C, Miller M, Fleming M. Mindfulness Meditation for Alcohol Relapse Prevention: a feasibility pilot study. *J Addict Med.* 2008;2:165–173.

Addiction Treatment Intervention: An Uncontrolled Prospective Pilot Study of Spiritual Self-Schema Therapy with Latina Women

Hortensia Amaro, PhD
Cielo Magno-Gatmaytan, MA
Michael Meléndez, MSW, PhD
Dharma E. Cortés, PhD
Sandra Arevalo, MA
Arthur Margolin, PhD

ABSTRACT. Spiritual Self-Schema (3-S) is a weekly 8-session, mindfulness-based, manual-guided, individual intervention targeting addiction and human immunodeficiency virus (HIV) risk behaviors that integrates cognitive behavioral strategies with Buddhist principles and clients' religious/spiritual beliefs. 3-S is efficacious for reducing drug use and HIV risk behaviors among mixed-gender, methadone-maintained outpatients. The study goal was to conduct a preliminary evaluation of 3-S therapy among urban, low-income Latinas ($n = 13$) in residential addiction treatment. Data gathered via in-person interviews (baseline, 8 and 20 weeks postentry) showed high rates of 3-S acceptability and positive changes in a number of outcomes relevant to recovery from addiction and to HIV prevention, including impulsivity, spirituality, motivation for change, and HIV prevention knowledge. The study findings are promising; however, a controlled study with longer follow-up is needed to rigorously assess the efficacy of 3-S therapy with Latinas in substance abuse treatment.

INTRODUCTION

Addiction treatment provides an important opportunity to introduce interventions aimed at decreasing the risk of human immunodeficiency virus (HIV) infection associated with drug use and unsafe sexual behaviors (1). There is an emerging interest in incorporating spirituality into addiction treatment (2), since spirituality, as a coping strategy, may play a protective role

Hortensia Amaro, Cielo Magno-Gatmaytan, Michael Meléndez, Dharma E. Cortés, and Sandra Arevalo are affiliated with the Institute on Urban Health Research, Bouvé College of Health Sciences, Northeastern University, Boston, Massachusetts, USA.

Michael Meléndez is also affiliated with Simmons College School of Social Work, Boston, Massachusetts, USA.

Arthur Margolin is affiliated with the Department of Psychiatry, Yale School of Medicine, Boston, Massachusetts, USA.

The manuscript was prepared with the support from the Bouvé College Research Grants Program, Northeastern University, and the US Department of Health and Human Services, Substance Abuse and Mental Health Administration, Center for Substance Abuse Treatment grant 1H79TI 14442-0 awarded to Dr. Hortensia Amaro. The authors also thank the program staff who assisted in the study implementation (Bethany Stuart, Brenda Marshall, and Rita Nieves) and the clients who participated in the study.

in physical and mental health (3). Spiritual Self-Schema (3-S) therapy, a manual-guided intervention delivered in 8 weekly individual sessions, incorporates clients' spiritual beliefs/religious faith. The 3-S framework is based on Buddhist philosophy and was chosen to accommodate a wide variety of theistic and nontheistic religious traditions and spiritual belief systems (3–5). The goal of 3-S therapy is to facilitate a cognitive shift in the client's predominant self-schema from the "addict self," with its associated scripts, action plans, and behaviors that can lead to the transmission of HIV and other infections (3, 6), to the "spiritual self" that is congruent with harm reduction and health promotion attitudes and behaviors (3, 6, 7). 3-S therapy is not solely a "talk-therapy," but also a practical, experiential therapy that helps clients become aware of their spiritual nature as a fundamental basis for ongoing growth and development as well as for preventive, health-oriented behavior. 3-S therapy is expected to improve an individual's spirituality, motivation to change, and HIV prevention knowledge, and to reduce impulsivity that is correlated with risky behaviors such as unprotected sex and drug use.

Examining the acceptability and promise of 3-S therapy with Latinas in treatment was undertaken for several reasons. First, HIV risk behaviors and HIV infection/acquired immune deficiency syndrome (AIDS) rate are disproportionately high among Latina drug users (8–10) and there is a need for effective interventions. Second, previous studies of 3-S therapy were limited to methadone-maintained outpatients, and thus issues of client acceptability and potential efficacy of 3-S therapy among Latina women in residential treatment have not been investigated. Lastly, the spiritual basis of 3-S therapy might make it particularly well suited for Latinas because spirituality has been identified as a powerful motivator for their recovery (11).

The objectives of this uncontrolled prospective pilot study were (1) to assess acceptability of 3-S therapy among Latinas as measured by participants' satisfaction, perceived credibility of the intervention, and perceived effects of the intervention on their addictive behaviors and sense of spirituality; and (2) to assess changes over time in participants' levels of impulsivity, spirituality, motivation to change drug use and HIV risk behaviors, and HIV prevention knowledge over the 20-week study duration. Because of the pilot nature of the study and the small sample size, we did not expect to detect statistically significant changes overtime.

METHODS

The study was conducted from October 2007 through March 2008 at Entre Familia, a program of the Boston Public Health Commission. Entre Familia is a gender- and culture-specific residential addiction treatment program for adult Latinas. The program provides long-term (6- to 12-month) integrated treatment for addiction and co-occurring mental health disorders (primarily depression, anxiety, and post-traumatic stress disorder). It has the capacity to house approximately 21 women and 40 of their children at any given time. The program is based on a bio-psycho-social trauma-informed model for the treatment of addiction (12). Standard services consist of a series of skill-based, manual-guided group therapy sessions based on cognitive-behavioral therapy and psychoeducational approaches and include individual counseling and psychotherapy, intensive case management, and supportive services. The treatment is gender and culture specific and is provided under a family-centered model of care.

Participants

All clients receiving services at Entre Familia, a Boston-based residential treatment program for adult Latinas, were candidates for inclusion in the study if they (1) had been enrolled in the residential treatment program for at least 2 weeks, (2) were fluent in English, and (3) had an interest in receiving a spirituality-focused therapy. There were no exclusion criteria.

The treatment agency staff informed clients about the study and obtained their permission to be contacted by a study interviewer who explained the study in detail. After the prospective participants agreed to participate in the study, the interviewer obtained signed consent forms prior to conducting the interview. The study protocol was approved by the Institutional Review Board of Northeastern University. The first 13 women who met the inclusion criteria and agreed to participate were enrolled. Participants were compensated with a $20 store voucher for their participation in each assessment.

Data reported in this study were obtained via in-person interviews conducted by a Latina researcher. Assessments were conducted at baseline, 8 weeks postentry, and 20 weeks postentry. In addition, data on the following background information were obtained via clinic records: substance abuse and mental health diagnoses, and history of physical, sexual, and emotional abuse.

Intervention

Participants received the 8 weekly 1-hour sessions of 3-S therapy delivered by a single doctoral-level Latino therapist with extensive experience in treatment of addiction and trauma in Latino populations. The clinician received intensive training in 3-S therapy, including a 3-day on-site comprehensive introduction by a certified 3-S therapy trainer and a 2-week advanced training on the delivery of each session from Dr. Arthur Margolin, 3-S therapy developer.

To ascertain fidelity of the study intervention, all sessions were videotaped and 20% were randomly selected for viewing and rating by the 3-S therapy developer, who also held weekly supervision conference calls with the therapist to review videotapes and clinical notes submitted on each client during each intervention session. The 3-S therapy developer's ratings showed high fidelity to the intervention manual for each session (3.5 on a scale from 0 to 4). Detailed information about the intervention, as well as the therapy manuals, is available on the 3-S Web site, www.3-S.us, under the "training" link.

Measures

Baseline Demographics and Clinical Characteristics

At the baseline interview, conducted by the research interviewer, demographic (age and years of education) and clinical characteristic measures were collected.

Addiction severity was measured using the Addiction Severity Index (ASI) composite scores for alcohol and drug addiction severity (13). Scores ranged from 0 (no symptoms) to 1.0 (highest severity) (13). The ASI is a widely used tool to evaluate problems of substance abusers. It demonstrated high interrater reliability (14) and has been used across different populations including homeless substance abusers (15) and substance abusers with mental illness (16). When the ASI was used with clients in a network of inner-city alcohol and drug abuse clinics, reliability scores were .84 for alcohol and .69 for drug addiction severity (17). Cronbach's alpha in the present study was .78 for alcohol and .68 for drug addiction severity.

Posttraumatic stress symptom severity was measured using the Symptom Severity Score (SSC), a subscale of the 49-item Posttraumatic Diagnostic Scale (PDS) (18). The SSC is a 17-item scale that assesses symptom severity from 0 ("not at all" or "only one time") to 3 ("5 or more times a week/almost always"). The SSC yields a total severity score (ranging from 0 to 51) reflecting the frequency of the 17 posttraumatic stress symptoms, with scores 1–10 indicating mild, 11–20 moderate, 21–35 moderate-to-severe, and 36–51 severe posttraumatic stress severity. SSC reliability tested in various racial/ethnic groups was high (Cronbach's alpha $>.90$) (18). Cronbach's alpha in the present study was .87.

Severity of mental health symptomatology was measured using the Global Severity Index (GSI) of the Brief Symptom Inventory (BSI) (19). GSI was used as a measure of general clinical distress. Using a 0 (not at all) to 4 (extremely) Likert scale, participants rated how much they were bothered by each of 18 mental health problems (symptoms) in the past 7 days, with pathology indicated by a T-score ≥ 63. BSI subscores for depression, anxiety, and somatization were also reported. Total scores for the GSI and BSI subscores range from 0 through 4, with higher scores indicating more severe mental health symptomatology. The GSI reliability tested with various racial/ethnic groups is high (Cronbach's alpha $>.90$) (19). Cronbach's alpha in the present study was .93.

119

Primary Outcomes

Acceptability of 3-S therapy was assessed with 3 measures. The first measure, the Participant's Post Intervention Satisfaction Questionnaire, asked participants to indicate how satisfied they were with the services they received during the intervention on a scale of 0 (not at all satisfied) to 10 (extremely satisfied) (4, 7). The second measure, the Treatment Credibility Scale (TCS) (3), assessed participants' confidence about the benefits of the intervention using 7 items with response values ranging from 0 (not at all) to 4 (extremely confident). The TCS was adapted by the developers of 3-S therapy from a scale developed for studies of acupuncture with reported Cronbach's alpha of .88 (20). The TCS score is the average of these 7 items, with a higher score indicating greater confidence. The TCS was administered at baseline and 8 weeks postentry. Cronbach's alpha in the present sample was .87. The third measure was the Post Treatment Questionnaire consisting of 7 items, using a 0 (not at all) to 10 (extremely) Likert scale. It asked participants how satisfied they were with 3-S therapy and how much it helped in reducing addiction and risk for HIV infection. The percentages of participants with positive perceived impact of the therapy were reported. The Participants' Post Intervention Satisfaction Questionnaire and the Post Treatment Questionnaire were used to measure intervention fidelity in a previous 3-S study but no reliability scores were reported (4, 7). In the present study, the reliability scores for the Participant's Post Intervention Satisfaction Questionnaire and the Post Treatment Questionnaire were Cronbach's alphas .83 and .98, respectively.

Secondary Outcomes

Impulsivity was assessed with the 30-item Barratt Impulsivity Scale—Revised (BIS-R), a widely used tool developed "to identify a set of impulsivity items that are orthogonal to a set of anxiety items" and "to define impulsiveness within the structure of related personality traits" (21). Response categories range from 0 (rarely/never) to 4 (almost always/always). A total score was computed by summing the items, with a higher score implying higher impulsiveness. Its internal consistency coefficients range from .79 to .83 among different populations of undergraduate students, prison inmates, substance abuse patients, and general psychiatric patients (21). Reliability was adequate (Cronbach's alpha .81) in the present study.

Spirituality was assessed using the Expression of Spiritual Qualities in Daily Life, a 10-item questionnaire that measured the following daily-life spiritual qualities: generosity, morality, renunciation, wisdom, effort, tolerance, truth, strong determination, loving kindness, and equanimity (6). Participants were asked to indicate "how much of the time you actually expressed this quality in your own life in the past week." Response categories ranged from 0 (not at all) to 4 (extremely). A mean score was computed with a higher score indicating higher spirituality. This measure was developed for and evaluated in a 3-S efficacy study with mixed-gender methadone participants in an outpatient setting and showed good reliability (Cronbach's alpha .89) (6), comparable to that found in the present study (.87).

Overall motivation to change drug use and HIV transmission–related behavior was assessed with a scale of 24 items that ranged from 0 (strongly disagree) to 4 (strongly agree). Higher scores indicate higher motivation. This measure was developed for and evaluated in a prior 3-S efficacy study with mixed-gender methadone participants in an outpatient setting in which reliability for the overall mean motivation to abstain from drug use and prevent HIV was adequate (Cronbach's alpha .84) (4). The reliability for overall mean motivation in this prior study was Cronbach's alpha .83. This measure has 3 subscales evaluating (1) motivation for abstinence, a 5-item instrument that measures motivation to abstain from drug use (Cronbach's alpha .78 in the present sample); (2) motivation vis-à-vis cognitive control, a 9-item instrument that measures perceived consequences of actions and ability for self control (Cronbach's alpha .6 in the present sample); and (3) motivation for HIV prevention and HIV transmission–related behaviors, a 10-item instrument that measures motivation for HIV prevention and HIV-related behaviors (Cronbach's alpha .41 in the present sample). To improve the reliability of the last 2 measures in our sample, we deleted 3 items in each. The final, 7-item measures showed improved Cronbach's alphas (.73 and .68, respectively).

HIV prevention knowledge was assessed with 20 multiple-choice questions evaluating knowledge of drug- and sex-related HIV transmission risks. This quiz is derived from the AIDS Information Sheet developed by the National Institute on Drug Abuse (22). A final score was computed as the percentage of correct answers. There is no reported reliability for this measure. In this study, the internal consistency KR-20 coefficient is high (>.90).

Statistical Methods

The size of the sample for this pilot study was determined based on the budget and time line available for the study.

Distributional data characteristics were assessed; data showed non-normal distribution, and nonparametric tests were used for analysis. Medians and ranges are reported for the outcome measures due to the nonparametric nature of the data. Friedman's analysis of variance was used to examine the longitudinal changes in scores during the whole study. Significance levels are reported at 2-tailed $P < .05$. Wilcoxon's signed-rank test examined changes between 2 time points. A Bonferroni correction was applied so all P values are reported at a $P < .0167$ level of significance. Because of the exploratory nature of the study, effect size r from the Wilcoxon's signed-rank test was calculated for the secondary outcomes. Effect size was interpreted as follows: small effect for $r < .3$; medium $r \geq .3$ but less than .5; large $r \geq .5$.

RESULTS

Retention and Treatment Attendance

Of the 13 subjects who completed baseline, 10 completed the 8- and 20-week postentry interviews. Analysis focuses on these 10 participants.

Seven of the 13 enrolled participants completed the intervention and all study assessments. Four were discharged from residential treatment prior to the study completion, but 3 of them completed all study assessments. Two other participants were withdrawn from the intervention due to psychopharmacological medication side effects (i.e., severe drowsiness and attention problems) that interfered with participation and did not complete study assessments. None of the participants, the therapist, or treatment staff reported any adverse or side effects from the intervention.

Baseline Demographics and Clinical Characteristics

Participants' ages ranged from 20 to 40 years (31 ± 7.5). Eleven of the 13 women were mothers with children under 18 years of age; the remaining were pregnant. The mean age of onset of alcohol use and drug use was 14 (± 2.9) and 15 (± 3.7), respectively. Ten women did not complete high school and had a history of homelessness. Eleven women had a history of incarceration and 9 had a history of arrests for drug-related offenses. All the women were Puerto Ricans.

All participants had a diagnosis of both substance use and mental health disorder (primarily depression and anxiety disorders), along with a history of sexual, physical, and/or emotional trauma. See Table 1 for a summary of the demographic and clinical profile of the sample.

Outcomes

Primary Outcomes: Treatment Acceptability

Mean 8-week postentry satisfaction scores (7.6 ± 2.2) indicated a rating between "moderately" and "extremely" satisfied.

Although treatment credibility scores increased across the 3 assessment periods, from "moderately" at baseline, to "very" credible at both 8 and 20 weeks postentry, these changes were not statistically significant. Medians and ranges are presented in Table 2.

After the 3-S intervention (8 weeks postentry), the average score on the 5 questions regarding the perceived effects of 3-S therapy was 2.7 (± 1.5) in a range from 0 to 4. The majority (70%) said that they felt "much closer" or "very much closer" to quitting drugs. In

TABLE 1. Baseline Demographic and Clinical Characteristics ($N = 13$)

Age, mean (SD)	31 (7.5)
Hispanic group, Puerto Rican, n %	13 (100)
No high school diploma, n (%)	10 (76.9)
Has history of homelessness, n (%)	10 (76.9)
Has history of incarceration, n (%)	11 (84.6)
Consumed alcohol in the past 30 days, n (%)	4 (30.8)
Used illegal drugs in the past 30 days, n (%)	8 (61.5)
Injected drugs in the past 30 days, n (%)	2 (15.4)
Alcohol Addiction Severity Index, score, mean (SD)	0.07 (0.1)
Drug Addiction Severity Index, score, mean (SD)	0.14 (0.1)
Posttraumatic stress symptomatology (PDS-SSC), total score, mean (SD)	34.33 (8.6)
Reexperiencing, subscale score, mean (SD)	9.92 (3.3)
Arousal, subscale score, mean (SD)	11.58 (3.4)
Avoidance, subscale score, mean (SD)	12.83 (4.8)
Mental health symptomatology (BSI-GSI), total score, mean (SD)	0.86 (0.9)
Depression, subscale score, mean (SD)	0.88 (0.9)
Anxiety, subscale score, mean (SD)	0.93 (0.9)
Somatization, subscale score, mean (SD)	0.78 (0.9)

addition, a majority reported that the following variables were affected "a lot" or "extremely" by participation in 3-S therapy: decreased craving for drugs (70%), increased experience and expression of spirituality (70%), experience of a shift from the addict self to the spiritual self (80%), and increased motivation to prevent the transmission of HIV (70%). Further, 60% reported that their drug use decreased "extremely" as a result of participation in 3-S therapy. The majority (80%) of participants indicated that they would like to continue 3-S therapy.

Secondary Outcomes: Impulsivity, Spirituality, Motivation, and HIV Prevention Knowledge

Results of Friedman's analysis of variance (ANOVA) showed statistically significant improvement over the course of the intervention (8 weeks) and at 20 weeks postentry in spirituality ($P < .05$), overall motivation to change drug use and HIV transmission–related behavior

($P < .05$), and HIV prevention knowledge ($P < .01$). Other measures showed trends suggesting improvement but these did not reach statistical significance.

Ancillary Analyses: Effect Size r from Wilcoxon's Signed-Rank Test

As shown in Table 3, results from pairwise comparison (Wilcoxon's test) showed statistically significant changes in HIV prevention knowledge at 8 ($P < .0167$) and 20 ($P < .0167$) weeks postentry compared to baseline. No other pairwise comparisons were statistically significant.

For impulsivity, calculations showed medium effect size at 8 weeks and small effect size at 20 weeks compared to baseline. For spirituality, we found a medium effect size at 8 weeks and no effect at 20 weeks compared to baseline. Overall motivation to change drug use and HIV transmission–related behavior showed medium effect sizes at both 8 and 20 weeks compared to baseline. Finally, for HIV prevention knowledge, we found large effect sizes at both 8 and 20 weeks compared to baseline. Results of the Wilcoxon test and the effect size r scores are summarized in Table 3.

DISCUSSION

This study was an uncontrolled prospective pilot study of the 3-S therapy with 13 Latinas. It assessed the acceptability of the 8-week individual 3-S intervention as gauged by participant's satisfaction, perceived credibility of the intervention, and perceived effects of the intervention on their addictive behaviors and sense of spirituality. Overall, participants were satisfied with the 3-S intervention. Postintervention satisfaction scores indicated that participants were "moderately" to "extremely" satisfied. Ratings on credibility of the therapy and participants' perceptions on the effects of 3-S therapy were positive and consistent with the high satisfaction ratings.

The study also assessed changes over time in participants' levels of impulsivity, spirituality,

TABLE 2. Results of Friedman's ANOVA Comparing Outcomes Across Measurement Points ($n = 10$)

Outcome measures	Baseline	8 weeks postentry	20 weeks postentry	χ_F^2	P
Treatment credibility, score, median (min–max)	2.0(1.1–3.9)	2.6(0.7–4.0)	2.9(1.0–4.0)	1.7	.433
Level of impulsivity, score, median (min–max)	73.5(65.0–106.0)	71.0(52.0–91.0)	73.5(51.0–91.0)	1.4	.500
Spirituality, score, median (min–max)	3.5(1.8–4.0)	3.8(2.6–4.0)	3.3(2.1–4.0)	6.2	.045
Overall motivation to change drug use and HIV transmission–related behavior, total score, median (min–max)	2.4(1.9–3.2)	2.8(2.2–4.0)	2.9(1.5–3.4)	6.2	.045
Motivation for drug abstinence, subscale score, median (min–max)	2.7(0.8–3.6)	3.0(2.0–4.0)	3.1(1.0–3.6)	1.7	.428
Motivation vis-à-vis cognitive control, subscale score, median (min–max)	2.6(1.7–3.4)	3.0(1.6–4.0)	2.7(1.7–4.0)	3.9	.139
Motivation for HIV prevention and decreased HIV-related behaviors, subscale score, median (min–max)	2.1(1.4–3.3)	2.6(1.7–4.0)	2.9(1.0–3.1)	5.0	.083
HIV prevention knowledge, total score, median (min–max)	57.5(45.0–85.0)	77.5(55.0–95.0)	82.5(60.0–95.0)	16.7	.001

motivation for abstinence from drug use, HIV risk behavior, and HIV prevention knowledge. Self-reported changes from baseline to 20 weeks postentry showed statistically significant changes in the levels of spirituality, motivation, and HIV prevention knowledge among participants. No significant changes were observed in impulsivity measures.

TABLE 3. Results of the Wilcoxon Test for Post Hoc Comparison and Intervention Effect Sizes ($n = 10$)

Outcome measures	Comparison time frame	t-statistic	z-score	P	r
Treatment credibility, score	Baseline–8 weeks postentry	11.0	−1.0	.326	−.2
	Baseline–20 weeks postentry	14.0	−1.4	.167	−.3
Level of impulsivity, score	Baseline–8 weeks postentry	7.5	−2.0	.041	−.4
	Baseline–20 weeks postentry	19.0	−0.4	.678	−.1
Spirituality, score	Baseline–8 weeks postentry	7.5	−1.8	.075	−.4
	Baseline–20 weeks postentry	22.0	−0.1	.953	.0
Overall motivation to change drug use and HIV transmission–related behavior, total score	Baseline–8 weeks postentry	10.0	−1.8	.074	−.4
	Baseline–20 weeks postentry	15.0	−1.3	.202	−.3
Motivation for drug abstinence, subscale score	Baseline–8 weeks postentry	7.5	−1.5	.141	−.3
	Baseline–20 weeks postentry	14.5	−0.5	.624	−.1
Motivation vis-à-vis cognitive control, subscale score	Baseline–8 weeks postentry	8.5	−1.7	.970	−.4
	Baseline–20 weeks postentry	8.0	−1.4	.159	−.3
Motivation for HIV prevention and HIV transmission-related behaviors, subscale score	Baseline–8 weeks postentry	11.5	−1.6	.103	−.4
	Baseline–20 weeks postentry	14.5	−0.9	.342	−.2
HIV prevention knowledge, total score	Baseline–8 weeks postentry	0.0	−2.8	.005	−.6
	Baseline–20 weeks postentry	0.0	−2.8	.005	−.6

Note. A Bonferroni correction was applied so all P values are reported at a $P < .0167$ level of significance.

Primary Outcomes: 3-S Intervention Acceptability

We found evidence indicating acceptability of 3-S therapy among this sample of Latinas in addiction treatment. Scores from the Treatment Credibility Scale and the Post Treatment Questionnaire indicated that the majority benefited from the intervention, found it acceptable and useful, and reported a desire to continue this form of therapy. These findings are consistent with reported high levels of acceptability in a previous 3-S therapy study with a different population (6). Latina participants in the current study found many of the spirituality-promoting aspects of 3-S therapy useful. 3-S therapy's use of visualization, mindfulness, cognitive reframing, and meditation practices were generally well received and appeared to be a good fit for this client population. Previous studies using these approaches with men and women, patients in the methadone maintenance program, reported similar findings (6, 23).

Secondary Outcomes: Potential Promise with Latina Women

We found a trend indicating a reduction in impulsivity over the course of the intervention period. However, at 20 weeks postentry, impulsivity returned to baseline values. It is possible that the effects faded over time or never took place. Controlled studies are needed to evaluate this issue.

The decrease in impulsivity over the course of intervention is consistent with the findings of another study of 3-S therapy that focused on impulsivity as an outcome (7). Analysis of baseline and 8-week postentry data in that study suggested that 3-S therapy not only increased spiritual practices that were antithetical to impulsivity but it also significantly reduced impulsivity scores compared to those of nonclinical samples.

Consistent with our findings, a previous 3-S therapy study found improvement in the frequency of spiritual qualities practice in daily life from baseline to 8 weeks postentry (3). As with impulsivity, in the present study, the return to baseline values at 20-week follow-up suggests

that these individuals may benefit from "booster sessions."

Findings of increased motivation to reduce high-risk behaviors and drug use throughout the present study are also consistent with findings of the previous studies of 3-S therapy (4, 7, 24).

In addition, HIV prevention knowledge increased significantly between baseline and 8 weeks postentry, and these improvements were maintained at 20 weeks postentry. Because the rates of HIV risk behaviors and HIV infection are disproportionately high among Latina drug users (9, 10), development of effective HIV prevention interventions is critical for this population. Although knowledge alone is not predictive of behavior change, it is an important first step because studies (25–27) have documented misconceptions and lack of accurate information regarding HIV prevention knowledge in this population. These educational gaps can undermine reduction of HIV-related high-risk behaviors.

Main limitations of this pilot study include the lack of a control group, small sample size, and a relatively short follow-up period. The choice of Latinas treated in residential settings as the studied population limits generalizability of our findings to Latinas in other treatment settings. Finally, the sample was comprised of Puerto Rican women and findings may differ for other Latina groups.

CONCLUSIONS

Findings from this pilot study suggest that 3-S therapy was well received by Latina women in residential treatment and may be a useful intervention for reducing impulsivity, increasing motivation for abstinence and spiritual practices, reducing high-risk behaviors, and increasing receptivity for HIV-prevention knowledge. Based on these findings, 3-S therapy warrants a controlled study in this clinical population.

REFERENCES

1. National Institute on Drug Abuse. *Principles of HIV Prevention in Drug-Using Populations*. Bethesda, MD: National Institute of Health; 2002.

2. Geppert C, Bogenschutz MP, Miller WR. Development of a bibliography on religion, spirituality and addictions. *Drug Alcohol Rev.* 2007;26:389–395.

3. Avants SK, Margolin A. Development of Spiritual Self-Schema (3-S) therapy for the treatment of addictive and HIV risk behavior: a convergence of cognitive and Buddhist psychology. *J Psychother Integrat.* 2004;14:253–289.

4. Margolin A, Beitel M, Schuman-Olivier Z, Avants SK. A controlled study of a spirituality-focused intervention for increasing motivation for HIV prevention among drug users. *AIDS Educ Prevent.* 2006;18:311–322.

5. Avants SK, Margolin A. *Spiritual Self Schema Therapy manual.* 2003. Retrieved August 5, 2007, from http://www.3-s.us/.

6. Avants SK, Beitel M, Margolin A. Making the shift from 'addict self to spiritual self.' Results from a stage I study of Spiritual Self Schema (3-S) therapy for treatment of addiction and HIV risk behavior. *Mental Health Religion Culture.* 2005;8:167–177.

7. Margolin A, Schuman-Olivier Z, Beitel M, Arnold RM, Fulwiler CE, Avants SK. A preliminary study of Spiritual Self-Schema (3-S+) therapy for reducing impulsivity in HIV-positive drug users. *J Clin Psychol.* 2007;63:979–999.

8. Center for Disease Control and Prevention. *HIV/AIDS Surveillance Report 18.* 2006. Available at: http://www.cdc.gov/hiv/topics/surveillance/resources/reports. Accessed September 19, 2008.

9. Kottiri BJ, Friedman SR, Neaigus A, Curtis R, Des Jarlais DC. Risk networks and racial/ethnic differences in the prevalence of HIV infection among injection drug users. *J Acquir Immune Defic Syndr.* 2002;30:95–104.

10. National Institute on Drug Abuse. Hispanics and drug abuse. NewsScan NIDA Addiction Research News (Feb). 2007. Available at: http://www.drugabuse.gov/newsroom/07/NS-2.html. Accessed September 11, 2008.

11. Arévalo S, Prado G, Amaro H. Spirituality, sense of coherence, and coping responses in women receiving treatment for alcohol and drug addiction. *Eval Program Plann.* 2008;31:113–123.

12. Amaro H, McGraw S, Larson MJ, López L, Nieves R, Marshall B. Boston Consortium of Services for Families in Recovery: a trauma-informed intervention model for women's alcohol and drug addiction treatment. *Alcohol Treat Q.* 2005;22:95–119.

13. McLellan AT, Kushner H, Metzger D, et al. The Fifth Edition of the Addiction Severity Index. *J Subst Abuse Treat.* 1992;9:199–213.

14. McLellan AT, Luborsky L, Cacciola J, et al. New data from the Addiction Severity Index: reliability and validity in three centers. *J Nerv Mental Dis.* 1985;173:412–423.

15. Argeriou M, McCarty D, Mulvey K, Daley M. Use of the Addiction Severity Index with homeless substance abusers. *J Subst Abuse Treat.* 1994;11:359–65.

16. Hodgins DC, El-Guebaly N. More data on the Addiction Severity Index: reliability and validity with the mentally ill substance abuser. *J Nerv Mental Dis.* 1992;180:197–201.

17. Leonhard C, Mulvey K, Gastfriend DR, Shwartz M. The Addiction Severity Index: a field study of internal consistency and validity. *J Subst Abuse Treat.* 2000;18:129–135.

18. Foa EB, Cashman L, Jaycox L, Perry K. The validation of a self-report measure of posttraumatic stress disorder: the Posttraumatic Diagnostic Scale. *Psychol Assess.* 1997;9:445–451.

19. Derogatis L. *Brief Symptom Inventory (BSI): Administration, Scoring and Procedures Manual,* 4th ed. Minneapolis: National Computer Systems; 1993.

20. Vincent C. Credibility assessments in trials of acupuncture. *Complement Med Res.* 1990;4:8–11.

21. Patton JH, Stanford MS, Barratt ES. Factor structure of the Barratt Impulsiveness Scale. *J Clin Psychol.* 1995;51:768–74.

22. National Institute on Drug Abuse. *Outreach/Risk Reduction Strategies for Changing HIV-Related Risk Among Injection Drug Users.* NIH Publication No. 94-3726. Rockville, MD: NIDA, 1994.

23. Simpson TL, Kaysen D, Bowen S, et al. PTSD symptoms, substance use, and vipassana meditation among incarcerated individuals. *J Trauma Stress.* 2007;20:239–249.

24. Beitel M, Genova M, Schuman-Olivier Z, Arnold R, Avants SK, Margolin A. Reflections by inner-city drug users on a Buddhist-based spirituality focused therapy: a qualitative study. *Am J Orthopsychiatry.* 2007;77:1–9.

25. Gómez C, Marín B. Gender, culture, and power: barriers to HIV-prevention strategies for women. *J Sex Res.* 1996;33:355–362.

26. Nyamathi A, Bennett C, Leake B, Lewis C, Flaskerud J. AIDS-related knowledge, perceptions, and behaviors among impoverished minority women. *Am J Public Health.* 1993;83:65–71.

27. Bernal G, Bonilla J, Bellido C. Ecological validity and cultural sensitivity for outcome research: issues for the cultural adaptation and development of psychosocial treatments with Hispanics. (Special Issue: Psychosocial Treatment Research.) *J Abnorm Child Psychol.* 1995;23:67–83.

Index

Page numbers in *Italics* represent tables.
Page numbers in **Bold** represent figures.
Page numbers followed by n represent endnotes.